TESTIMONIALS

"The book is not just another ER scene the story is real and alive, and it has a HEART. Anyone that reads the book will come away a better person being prepared and ready to face the world and its many challenges."

— Wilma Brown – IN

"This book is brutal. This book is funny and most importantly; this book is packed with heart from front to back. A sick man with the strength of 10 men, drug deals gone bad, gang bangers with no fear. Sex-crazed nurses. One man doing everything in his power to save lives, while at the same time, trying to stay out of the line of fire. This is good stuff."

— Mark Edward Marston –
Stillwater Gazette Newspaper – MN.

"This book has a making of a real live TV show."

— J.D. Inman – CA

"To really know what goes on in the inner-city rescuing people, this book gives a very inciteful preview."

— G. Robinson – PA

"Hats off to the Paramedics who risk their lives to save others. Johnson's experiences give me a better appreciation of our men and women in action."

— M.P. Roayster – WI

D1628800

"You can't put this book down. The action is non-stop."

– McDougal – GA

"The experiences Mr. Johnson shares in his book are exceptional for Paramedics. They are the real unsung heroes. Thumbs up for this well written book!"

– K. James – Mira Mesa, CA

The Sirens Never Stop!

True Stories and Experiences As Told
By
David Johnson

XULON PRESS

Xulon Press
2301 Lucien Way #415
Maitland, FL 32751
407.339.4217
www.xulonpress.com

Cover Design by: Anthony Henson
Editors: Mary Brown and Matthew J. Key
Contributing Editors: Mark Berriman and John Hardy
Copy Editing: Kelli Manion
First Edition – 2005, MN
Publisher: Matthew J. Key – Five Star Publishing – MN, CA

Paperback ISBN-13: 978-1-6628-6902-0
Ebook ISBN-13: 978-1-6628-6903-7

DEDICATION

This book is dedicated to all the medics that I had the pleasure of working with, those who taught me and those who learned from me.

I would also like to express my thanks to my wife and family for allowing me to take the time away from them to finish this project.

I want to thank my parents who always believed in me. They were my rock through all my turbulent years. I want to give a special thanks to my dad who constantly encouraged me to finish my book.

Last, but not least, I want to thank all my special friends who have been very supportive. I couldn't have done it without you.

I want to thank a very special co-writer, Mary Chris Brown, for the many hours that you spent with me rewriting my book. I could not have done it without you.

My last dedication goes to my best friend and longtime buddy and publisher, Matt Key, who was the first one to inspire me that I should put my experiences in a book.

ACKNOWLEDGMENTS

Why did I write this book? After 20 years of experiences in being involved in the emergency field, I just wanted to tell my side of the story. The uncut version of what an inner-city paramedic goes through in Gary, Indiana.

I must give credit to some of the best people I have worked with. Number one must be my partner and best friend, Russell Hayes.

Just to name a few great paramedics I had the pleasure of working with, they include Richard Spence, Albert Reese, Paulette, Greg Watkins, Kim Roscoe, Rochelle Hughes, Geraldine, Louise, Mike, Teddy, Bernard Henderson, Heavy D, Milt Jackson, and Sam Bruno.

Special thanks to Matt Cannefax and John Muller – Lakeview Hospital EMS – from Stillwater, Minnesota for their contribution to this book.

TABLE OF CONTENTS

Chapter 1   The Early Days 1

Chapter 2   Where It All Began 7

Chapter 3   The Emergency Room 19

Chapter 4   Fear of the Dead 31

Chapter 5   Code Seven. 39

Chapter 6   How I Became A Paramedic 49

Chapter 7   Now That I Have Made It – What's Next? 73

Chapter 8   A Night To Remember 91

Chapter 9   Now I Hit the Streets 99

Chapter 10   Working With Russ and Lashawn 115

Epilogue   Where Are They Now? 143

About the Author. 145

INTRODUCTION

What is it like to work in an urban community where crime runs rampant, and drugs and gangs are everywhere.

This is an example of our typical day. We would start the morning out trying to eat breakfast and end up on an ambulance run looking at someone who had just blew his head off. For lunch we would be working on auto accidents victims so bad they had to be cut out of the auto with limbs either missing or barely hanging on. Then as dinnertime rolled around, we would find ourselves running back and forth on stabbings, more gunshot wounds, and full cardiac arrests. As if that wasn't enough, to top things off we would get a call at 3 a.m. or 4 a.m. in the morning only to find someone who wanted an ambulance because the cab was too slow, and they wanted to go and visit a relative.

Yes, my 20 years as a paramedic have been jam-packed with every kind of story imaginable. When I first started working on the streets, I found out that my biggest job wasn't how to treat emergencies, but how to stay alive. When you read my story, you are going to find humor, excitement, sadness, love, passion, and more.

This book is not fiction; these are actual events that really happened. The names have been changed to protect people's right to autonomy. But if you have ever wondered what some paramedics go through in the inner city, this is the book to read. **Warning: Some of the material may be very graphic in detail, but I want you** *to read what I saw.* I will say this has been an experience I'm happy I didn't miss. So, fasten your seat belts and hold on. This is going to be quite a ride because *The Sirens Never Stop!*

CHAPTER 1
THE EARLY DAYS

IN THE EARLY DAYS IT WAS NOT UNCOMMON TO hear, "Hurry Russ, put an airway in the man's mouth and start CPR on that guy over there. LaShawn, grab those 4x4s and put pressure on this bleeder! Where is that other ambulance? Boy, this is a bad scene!" There was an accident on the expressway. Four cars and a semi-truck are involved. Suddenly one of the cars bursts into flames. There are three children trapped in the car with their mother. The screams are getting louder and louder. One fireman rushed over with the hose and started putting water on the car. The other firemen worked with the Jaws of Life trying to get the door open to free the family. Suddenly someone yells, "We're in! We're in!" As I looked over my shoulder, another ambulance had just arrived. I gave a big sigh of relief. We worked for the next 30 minutes trying to save as many as we could.

You see, when people are trapped, and cars are mangled, it takes time to try to get them out safely. Whether we triumph or fail, we still must keep a clear head because there is always the next run. You must get ready. You must be ready.

I remember when life wasn't so fast paced in this little steel town. I grew up back in the 1950s and the 60s in Gary, Indiana. Gary is a steel town and naturally almost everyone worked in one of the steel mills. My father was one of those workers. Life was easy-going back then. The kids would be playing cricket in the streets. To play this game you set up five to six cans in a row. The pitcher would go to the opposite end of the street about 20 feet away and roll a rubber ball at the cans. The batter would stand in front of the cans and try to hit the ball with a stick. If you missed, the ball would knock one or more cans down. Now the batter and pitcher would switch positions. The other kids would be playing basketball. Some would be shooting marbles. This is a game where the kids clear off a place in the sand and put their marbles in a circle. Then they would shoot a marble at the marbles in the circle trying to knock them out of the circle. The ones you knock out are the ones you get to keep. Sometimes you may win a bag full of marbles. There were so many harmless games we played back then. It was just a lot of fun to be around at that time.

Suddenly I felt this hand on my shoulder and the voice said, "Hey Doc. I think this man is dead. We have tried everything, but nothing has worked so far." I looked up, it was one of the other medics who came to assist. Whenever there is major trauma, you should call for assistance. The dispatcher will send extra manpower to the scene. Notice that I was called Doc. That was the nickname they gave me. You will see later how I got that name. Russ and I immediately started CPR on this man. He was the driver of the semi-truck. We believe that he had a heart attack, thereby causing the accident. The witnesses stated that he was swerving and ran into the other cars.

My partner, Russ, put the man on the heart monitor and gave me a strip of his heart rhythm. His EKG rhythm showed a straight line. This rhythm shows that the heart is not beating.

We are getting ready to defibrillate this man." This means that we are going to administer a certain amount of Jules from a defibrillator that will shock the patient's heart. I told everyone,

2

"Stand back! I'm getting ready to shock the patient." If anyone is touching any part of the patient, they will receive the shock also. I administered the shock. The patient's whole body jumped. Then I looked at the cardiac monitor and noticed the patient now had a cardiac rhythm. It was what we call in medical terms, a Brady rhythm. A Brady rhythm is a slow rhythm. The normal heart beats 60-80 beats per minute. Anything under 60 is considered a Brady Rhythm, but this is good. Any medic will take this kind of rhythm in a full arrest situation. The reason being is that we can give medications to increase the rate of the rhythm. This is not a dying heart rhythm.

A paramedic should always give his best effort to save a life because you only have one. That is why we are always ready ... always prepared.

Now that we had a heart rhythm on this man, I checked his pulse. "Yes! He has a pulse!" His heart is beating again, and he is now trying to breathe on his own. Suddenly, I heard LaShawn calling me. "Hey Doc! Hey Doc! I can't stop the bleeding on this man in the red car!" I told the other paramedic that came to assist to take over and expedite this man to the hospital, stat. This means transport right away to the hospital emergency room. I said, "Tell the hospital ER that he was a full arrest, but we got him back." I rushed over to assist LaShawn. When we are working in a situation like this, we are trained to do quick assessments to ascertain the most urgent and life-threatening injuries. I noticed part of the dashboard had been pushed in on his legs all the way up to his thigh. The sharp metal in the dash had punctured an artery in his thigh. This is very, very serious. That specific artery, which is called the femoral artery, can deplete a person's blood supply in a matter of minutes. To get to the man, LaShawn had to climb through the window on the passenger's side of the car.

I told her, "Keep pressure on that artery, I'm coming in." Once I climbed in, I immediately reinforced her pressure bandage with more bandages. I told her to set me up with an IV of Ringers Lactate. This is a volume expander fluid that you give people when they are losing blood. I started the IV and started pushing fluids. The one thing that I liked about LaShawn, and Russ is I never had to tell them to do the little things that EMTs do for patients. Things like giving oxygen and taking vitals. LaShawn had all those bases covered. I said, "LaShawn, what is his blood pressure?" She said, "90/60." The patient's color was very pale, and he was very lethargic. I called Russ and told him to have the bed ready so when the firemen free this man from the car with the Jaws of Life, we can expedite him to the hospital right away.

The other people in the other cars that were involved only had minor injuries and the medics that came to assist took care of them.

Suddenly the fireman says, "He's free!" We put him on the spine board. A cervical collar was applied to his neck. We put him on a short board and pulled him out and on to a long board. This is necessary for any car accident to help protect the patient's spine. Away to the ambulance we go. Once loaded, I called the hospital. We have a radio setup so that we can talk directly to the hospital just by picking up the bio-phone. I called and said, "Medic 100 to the trauma center." They answered and said, "Go ahead medic 100." I said, "I'm coming in with a 40-year-old male, approximately 180 pounds, no medical history, not on any medication, who was involved in a collision, semi versus car. The patient had the dash pushed in on the left thigh, puncturing the femoral artery. We initiated code 1 (airway breathing and circulation). We also started an IV of Ringers and ran it wide open. The patient's vitals are as follows: Blood pressure 90/60, pulse 140, respirations 32, color pale, skin cool and moist, lungs clear, level of consciousness, patient is lethargic but responsive, pupils equal and reactive to light. Second set of vitals, after 500cc of ringers had been infused, are as follows: Blood pressure 110/80, pulse 120, and respirations 28. This patient is a class 4 trauma that will probably need surgical intervention. Our ETA (estimated time of arrival) is five minutes."

On our arrival to the hospital the ER was ready for us. They had already contacted surgery and plans were made to get the patient to surgery ASAP. While I was writing my report, Russ and LaShawn were replenishing the equipment we used. The ER doctor came over to us and said, "I just want to tell you guys that you did a good job out there. I checked the other victims, especially the ones trapped in the burning car. They got away with just minor burns. The quick intervention of the firemen helped." I asked the doctor about the man who was in full arrest. He said, "They rushed him to intensive care and his prognosis looks good."

As I sat and wrote my report, I couldn't help but think how far I had come from where I started. As a young man growing up in this small city, all I aspired to do when I got out of school was get a job in the mill like my dad. Not once did I ever envision that I would be saving people's lives.

When I came out of school in 1968, it was the height of the Vietnam War. Every young man of age was concerned about the draft. My family was very religious. I was brought up in a Christian home. In fact, I wanted to be a minister. So, I applied to the draft board for a minister's classification but was denied. They started the draft lottery in 1969. Everyone who received a high lottery number was sure to be drafted into the military. My lottery number was 780. Those whose numbers were 500 and up were considered high. Most of the time when you mention lottery today, people think about money. But this lottery didn't represent money, it represented lives. If your lottery number was pulled back, then all you were going to get was a free trip to the rice patties. Your prize would be an AK47 rifle strapped to your back. Everyone would know if you won the big prize. This would be the case if you managed to get out with your life or a piece of it anyway.

Under normal circumstances in a lottery, if your number were high, you would be jumping for joy. It was a sure sign that you were going to win something. Sad to say, at that turbulent time, it was the last thing you wanted.

I remember my good friend, Adelle Sneed. We went to school together. Everyone knew Adelle. He always had this big boom box radio he carried on his shoulders wherever he went. He was a nice quiet guy who loved music. Well, Adelle hit the jackpot. He got sent to Vietnam as soon as he graduated. Several months later we learned that Adelle was fatally wounded. I wonder if the medics who dedicated their lives to saving people, like I have, were there to help poor Adelle.

There were so many of our classmates and friends coming home in body bags. It was like sheep going to the slaughter. I didn't go to Vietnam due to my moral beliefs. I was taught to be non-violent. I ended up being sentenced by a judge to do two years of civilian duty. This would entail working anywhere that provides a service to help people. I chose to go to the hospital. And…this is where it all began.

CHAPTER 2

WHERE IT ALL BEGAN

THE 1960S AND 70S WERE TURBULENT TIMES FOR young men in America. There were so many issues going on in this country. There was a general feeling of hopelessness. Groups were springing up everywhere. Some were pro war, and some were anti-war. It was a time of great polarization. People were either hawks or doves. When they took either position, they were willing to give their lives for their stand. The assassination of John F. Kennedy and Martin Luther King Jr. only made things worse. Then came the riots that burned and destroyed major cities. It was the climax of human frustration at a system that failed to meet people's expectations socially, politically, and economically.

In 1972, the courts sentenced me to do two years of civilian duty. I got a job at Lutheran General Hospital. Prior to that, I worked in the steel mill in Gary, Indiana. To perform this duty, I had to work at Lutheran General full time. So, the mill gave me a two-year leave of absence. Most of the guys were on their way to boot camp. Little did I know that I was on my way to 'butt' camp.

I spent many hours carrying bedpans and cleaning patients. Just like the guys in Vietnam who had never been in the hills and the rice patties and could not speak the Vietnamese language, I was in foreign territory too. The hospital had its own language. For instance, the nurse told me to go and get the I's and O's. I knew it wasn't tick tack toe, but what it meant I had no idea. I found out this was how they measure the patient's intake and output. This entailed checking how much they drank and dumping their urine bottle. The nurse also asked me if the patient had a BM or had the patient voided. I knew about M&M's, but not BM. This meant did the person have a bowel movement and had they urinated. As you can see, just like the guys in Vietnam lost in the rice patties, I was lost at Lutheran General Hospital.

Lutheran General Hospital was the second oldest hospital in this city. It was a big brick complex that always seemed to be in the process of remodeling or expanding. A lot of the units in the hospital were old with six or seven bed wards. The beds either had wood or metal frames. Most of the nurses were older women who wore uniforms with aprons in the front and bonnets on their heads. The uniforms matched their attitudes; old fashioned, no nonsense and no sense of humor.

To get this job, I had to take a class to become a Nursing Assistant. My instructor was Ms. Livingston. She was a short, thin Puritan-looking elderly lady who wore a bonnet perched on top of a bun on her head. Not one strand of her hair was out of place.

Have you ever had a staff sergeant that did not like you? For some reason, she just didn't like me. The courts sentenced me to work for two years. Ms. Livingston knew this. But the kicker was, I had to pass her class to get the job. As you guessed it, we bumped heads. Boy did we bump heads! Like the boys in the military going through basic training, I also had to walk the chalk line in hospital boot camp. She watched me like a mother hawk. How is it that men can listen and take orders from their mother but hate the orders coming from another woman? She told the class that if your head nurse decides to chew you out, you must stand there and take it. She also said you are not allowed to say anything back. Now, I had to disagree with her on this one. Even though I knew when I did, the boom would be lowered on me. I told her no one has the right to chew you out just because they are having a bad day. Just like in the military, if you say anything to disagree with the sergeant, you are going to end up digging a hole, ironing clothes, running, or doing pushups until you drop. Well, I was on official KP (kitchen patrol duties that you get if the military wants to punish a soldier), and there was no room for error, otherwise I was going to get kicked out. I worked extremely hard to make a perfect bed. I caught her many times in my room trying to pull my sheets apart. In the class, when we took a test, I had to write an essay just to get her to accept my answer. But I passed basic training. What's the expression, you are in the army now? Now I am a staff member of the Lutheran General Hospital. Little did I know that my battle had just begun?

Once you finish class, they assign you to a floor to work on. I had never been around sick people before. This was a new experience for me. I was now introduced to my head nurse, Mrs. Draper. She was at the opposite end of the spectrum from Ms. Livingston. She was fresh out of nursing school with a master's degree in Nursing. Mrs. Draper was a tall (approximately 5'9" tall), very fair complexion African American woman with a medium build. In comparison to the other head nurses, she was young, about 23 or 24 years old. She weighed approximately 170 pounds. I was so happy to get away from Ms. Livingston, only to find out I had just inherited her daughter, Mrs. Draper. They were not related but they both had the same no-nonsense attitude. I really felt that Mrs. Draper tried to over-compensate her firmness because she was young. My other theory was she and Ms. Livingston attended the same school of nursing and part of their training included no smiling, no personality, and no people skills. I'm sure they passed with flying colors.

Let me give you an example of what I'm talking about. One day, one of the nurse's aides received a phone call from her babysitter, telling her that her baby was very sick. They wanted her to come and get her child. The young lady went to Mrs. Draper and told her what the situation was and that she needed to leave. Mrs. Draper told her that she would have to find someone else to go and attend to her child. She had a job to do, and her patients also needed her. She informed the nurse's aide that she was not going to get permission to leave. I'm sure I don't have to tell you what the nurse's aide told her to do with her job. This is how she dealt with her staff.

I don't know what Ms. Livingston told her about me, but she tried to make my life miserable. For instance, I was given the worst patients that we had on the floor. All my patients were completes. These are patients who are bed ridden and cannot do anything for themselves. I was given eight to 10 patients a day. She would also chew me out if I was not finished by the end of the shift. Being the only man on my floor required me to stop many times to help the other ladies with their heavy patients. Also, the male orderlies had to go all over the hospital to put in Foley Catheters. These were Teflon tubes that were inserted into the penis of the men who had a problem urinating or in the elderly men who kept wetting the bed. Yes, my days were full. I can still hear her voice, "Johnson, you are not leaving until you finish these patients, and I am not paying you overtime." By the way I only made $2 an hour.

Working in the hospital was not a straight shift, you had to work swing turn. That was days, evenings, and midnights. When I got on the other shifts, I just knew it was going to be so much better since I was not going to be around Mrs. Draper. In the military, even when the captain is not there the sergeants make sure you carry out the assigned tasks. The hospital did not have sergeants, but they had charge nurses and boy did they crack that whip. I can still hear them, "All right Johnson, let's go! Get some gloves and some towels so we can clean up every patient on this floor. Just because you are not on days does not mean that you get to take it easy. We are going to work tonight." I soon realized that I might as well settle in and go along for the ride. Bucking against the system was only going to make things worse for me.

Well things might have started off kind of rough, but it wasn't all bad. I can recall so many funny moments when I thought I would never get through laughing.

I walked into this four-bed ward one day and this little old man, Mr. Crisps, was picking things out of the air and putting them in his mouth. He was a thin, sandy, gray-haired man in his 80s who was confused. I said, "Mr. Crisp, what are you doing?" He said, "Eating grapes." I said, "Really," in a sarcastic tone of voice. I didn't see anything in the air, especially not grapes. One of the other patients in the room said, "Why did you all put me in here with this crazy man?" I walked over to his bed and observed him. He was firmly convinced that there were some grapes in front of him, but there was nothing there. I said, "Are they good?" He said, "They are delicious. Would you like some?" I said, "Sure." He said, "Try the green ones. They don't have any seeds in them." The other men in the room said, "That old fool is nuts." I laughed it off and left the room.

But later that evening we heard some screams coming from the room across the hall from Mr. Crisp's room. We ran down there as fast as we could. Mr. Crisp had gotten up to use the bathroom. He had taken off his hospital gown and was wandering around nude trying to find his bed. He had gone across the hall into a room occupied by this little elderly lady, Miss Flowers. Miss Flowers had just gotten up to go to the bathroom only to come out and find a naked man in her bed. We said, "Mr. Crisp, what are you doing?" He said, "I just got in my bed and this woman is trying to share it with me! She can't get into my bed; my wife would not like that!" We had to take Mr. Crisp across the hall and put him in his correct bed. We tried to comfort Miss Flowers by giving her some coffee to calm her down.

We went back to the nurse's station and had a big laugh. Then, 15 minutes later we noticed the call light from Mr. Crisp's room flashing like crazy at the nurse's station. We ran down to the room. The other men in the room yelled, "Get this crazy old man out of here! He is throwing his BM across the room into our beds!" Mr. Crisp was sitting there looking like the cat that ate the canary. He said, "I'm not bothering these guys. They keep picking at me." We had to restrain Mr. Crisp's hands so that the guys could get some rest.

Two weeks passed and I am back on the day shift with my friend Mrs. Draper. Well today proved to be an exciting day. In the hospital setting to save lives you must work together as a team. You should be committed to do whatever it takes medically to save the patient's life. I was committed to that philosophy until I saw this.

They gave a lot of classes to teach the nurses what to do in full-arrest situations. The nurse's aides were told if we witnessed a full arrest (that means if the patient's heart stops beating or they stop breathing), go to the first telephone we get to and push "O" for the operator. Tell them you have a Code Blue and what room it's in. Then the operator will announce the code blue over the intercom. The nurses were trained to respond right away. The first person in the room would immediately start mouth-to-mouth resuscitation. Yes, back then we were doing mouth-to-mouth resuscitation. The next person in the room was to start chest compressions. They were to keep this going until the Code Blue team came to take over. This was a team of nurses with the doctor specially trained in full-arrest situations.

I was in the room taking care of this man, Mr. Smith. He had just finished his breakfast. He was a large man with a huge abdomen. He had brown, straight hair and blue eyes. It was obvious from his size and the amount of food on his tray that he loved to eat. Most people don't particularly like hospital food, but Mr. Smith would ask for seconds. This specific day, Mr. Smith was eating so fast, he choked! He started to vomit and suddenly he fell back in the bed and stopped breathing! This incident scared me. I said to myself, "This is a Code Blue." I ran to the phone and said, "Code Blue, Code Blue room 236." Remember, I told you the man had vomited and the first person in the room was to start mouth-to-mouth. Guess who the first person was to come into the room. You guessed it, Mrs. Draper!

Mrs. Draper immediately grabbed a towel and wiped the man's mouth. Right at that time the assistant head nurse, Mrs. Aaronson, came in. Mrs. Draper told her, "I'll do chest compressions and you give mouth-to-mouth. I watched the assistant head nurse blow and blow into this man's mouth. Not once did I hear Mrs. Draper tell her the man had vomited. Now you know I could not keep that a secret. The Code Blue team came and took over. Poor Mr. Smith didn't make it.

The assistant head nurse went to the utility room to wash her hands. I walked in behind her and asked her tactfully, "Who is supposed to give mouth-to-mouth in a Code Blue situation?" Her reply was, "The first person on the scene." I told her that I was in the room with the man, and I called the Code Blue. I also told her the patient vomited before he arrested, and Mrs. Draper was the first one to come into the room. She knew the man had vomited.

She wiped his mouth and told you to give mouth-to-mouth, but she never told you that the man vomited.

Mrs. Aaronson immediately ran to the sink and started to rinse her mouth out. I thought I would never get through laughing. She went out and grabbed Mrs. Draper by her arm and spun her around so that they were face to face. She was screaming as she told her, "As long as you live don't you ever do that again! If I had to do mouth-to-mouth, you could at least inform me the patient has vomited." She added several expletives dilative stating what she thought of her and describing her unprofessional conduct. She stated in emphatic terms, "I am writing this up because you didn't follow protocol." Mrs. Draper's face was flushed. All the color was gone. Her eyes were bucked as a deer staring in a headlight. I know in the back of her mind she was wondering who told. She was so embarrassed and totally caught off guard. The onlookers were applauding. I led the cheer in my heart. I knew that if she knew I was the one who told, I would be dead meat.

In 1972, there was a break in at Watergate by the Republican Party that set the stage for a drastic change in American government. While the scene of the world was changing, I was as well. Most of the young men that were sent to Vietnam had no prior experience in hand-to-hand combat. They had to get extensive training to fight in the war. When I think about my situation, I was thrown into Lutheran General Hospital without any training on how to deal with all those women.

When I speak about hand-to-hand combat, let me give you an example of what I mean. One day, one of the nurse's aides came to me and said, "Johnson, we need you to help us with a patient in one of the private rooms down the hall." I said, "I'll be there in just a minute." I had no idea that the patient in that room had been discharged. It was about eight to 10 nurses and nurse's aides waiting in that room for me to come in. Remember, I told you that there weren't many men that worked in the hospital. They had decided they were going to have some fun with me. When I walked into the room, they immediately grabbed me by the collar, threw me down on the bed, closed the door, cut the lights off and everyone piled on top of me. I know you are thinking this is most men's fantasy. But the only thing that I could think of was, if Mrs. Draper walked into this room, I'm going to be the first one she fires. I couldn't afford to lose this job. If I did, the courts would send me anywhere in the USA where they had an opening. This would require me to take my family and move. Financially, I could not afford to do that. I'm begging these girls to get off me. They were kissing me, pulling on me, laughing, giggling, and having a great time. Somehow, I managed to get free. I broke out of that room looking like I'd been in World War III. Wouldn't you know it! Who do I run into but Mrs. Draper! She says, "Johnson, what in the world have you been doing?" I said, "Mrs. Draper, I know I look a mess but it's because I'm working so hard trying to get through." She said, "Go fix yourself up before you go back around those patients, you look a mess."

When I came to Lutheran General Hospital, I was a happily married man. I had only been married about a year and a half. You see, I got married right out of high school. I never had a lot of girlfriends. I didn't have a lot of experience working with women. The only people I had worked with were men. They would invite me out on dates and to their parties, but they specified, come by yourself. The flirting was endless. But I was as green as any apple in spring, and they knew it. They were always saying, "Johnson, you are too nice. We got to show you how to be a bad boy." My reply was, "No thanks, I'm fine the way I am."

I found out that even at my best, my best wasn't good enough. Not long after that, one of the nurse's aides came to me. The look on her face told me right away that something was seriously wrong. She said, "Johnson, can I speak to you for a minute." I said, "Sure, what is the problem?" She said, "I'm kind of embarrassed to tell you this, but last night when I was making love to my husband, I made a mistake and called your name." Remember, I told you about the look on her face. Now, that look is on my face. I might have been naïve, but not that naïve. I said, "Are you crazy! You must be trying to get me killed! Why would you do something stupid like that?" She said, "I don't know. I've always had this crush on you, and I just let myself get carried away!" I said, "Well there are a lot of men out there with my name. Maybe he won't suspect it was me." She said, "I think he'll suspect it's you because I talk about you all the time. I told him how much fun we have on the floor." This woman has really spoiled my day.

To show you how serious this was, I was off the next day; the girl's husband came to the floor to see me. As soon as he asked for me, the other nurse's aides came to my rescue. They pulled him into the office and let him have it. The hospital grapevine had carried this story, so all the girls on the floor knew about it almost as soon as I did.

They told him that I was a real nice young man. They also enlightened him of the fact that there were lots of ladies on the floor trying to get me. They said, "So far no one had succeeded." The ladies asked him a question that really embarrassed him. They said, "Why do you think he wants your wife; she is not that attractive. What she told you was her fantasy and not his. So, you need to go home and deal with your wife." The ladies said he was so embarrassed he left. We never heard anything about it again. But rest assured, I kept my distance from her.

Working on the floor was OK but I was getting bored, and I was getting tired of smelling BM and urine. I'm the kind of guy who needs excitement. I need something to challenge me. One of my good friends, Sam, worked in the Emergency Room and he encouraged me to come down to the ER and work. He was telling me how exciting it was. So, after working a year on the floor, I transferred to the Emergency Room. Now the excitement begins.

CHAPTER 3

THE EMERGENCY ROOM

HAVE YOU EVER BEEN IN A PLACE WHERE EVERY-thing seems to be moving, including the pictures on the wall? My first day in the ER was an eye opener. Never in my life have I witnessed so much chaos. People were dragging folks in. The police were dragging people out. People were fighting in the hallway. There were no private booths. The room was wide-open, maybe a curtain to separate the beds if the patients hadn't torn them down. Patients on the beds were screaming. Doctors were shouting out orders and the nurses were running like crazy. There was blood everywhere! One mother was shouting, "My baby is not breathing!" Another was screaming, "My son has been shot!" Another was saying, "My mother needs something for pain!" Others were shouting, "When are we going to see a doctor!" The doctors were shouting, "Bring me some sponges! I need oxygen on this patient over here! Someone set me up a suture tray! Is there anyone working in this place outside of me!" I quickly learned that the ER takes no prisoners. It was every man for himself.

The doctors would tell me to go and get a lot of things. The patients were asking me for things. People were pulling at my uniform wanting to fight. No one stopped to ascertain that I was new. I didn't know the front door from the back door. To them, you were either a part of the solution or a part of the problem. If you wanted excitement, the ER was the place to be. I'm sure you have heard the expression, 'Be careful what you wish for, it might come true.' I think this time I bit off more than I could chew. That night, while in bed, I found myself fighting people in my sleep. The ER was not for the squeamish. I soon found out the key to working in the ER is having knowledge of where everything is.

Dr. Westano was a little short, bald, medium-build man with no patience. He was well-dressed with an immaculately scrubbed, clean look. If his white jacket got one spot of blood on it, he would immediately change to another. He looked at me on my first day and said, "Who are you?" In return I said, "I'm the new orderly." He said, "What is your name?" I said, "Dave Johnson." He said, "OK Johnson bring me a hemostat." This is an instrument made like a pair of scissors, only the end looks like a pair of needle-nosed pliers. It is used to clamp off blood vessels that are bleeding. At the time, I didn't know a hemostat from a paper clip. I stood there looking at him and he said, "What are you waiting for a priest! The patient will be dead if I don't get one soon!" My buddy Sam saved me. He ran and gave Dr. Westano the hemostat. Sam was good. He was about 25 years old, 5'8" tall and approximately 165 pounds, with a nice muscular build. Sam was a black belt in karate. He worked out all the time. Sam always greeted everyone with a smile. He was a very pleasant person to be around. All the doctors loved Sam because he really knew the ER.

Dr. Westano said, "Johnson, bring me some catgut." At the time he was suturing an open wound. My reply was, "Doc, where in the world am I going to find some cat-guts and why would you want to put that in a wound?" I thought he would never get through laughing. He was doubled over. His face was flushed. The nurses had tears in their eyes from laughing so hard. He said, "No you idiot! Catgut is a suture that we use to close deep wounds."

Then he looked at the nurses and said, "Where in the world did you get this retarded kid?" They said, "Doc, he is just new. He will be OK." I can't tell you how embarrassed I was. It was at that point I made a concerted effort to learn procedures, the equipment, and the names of all the supplies used. Eventually, each day \got progressively easier. I was beginning to really enjoy the fast pace of the ER. The staff must work all three shifts because the ER is open 24 hours. After my second month, they felt I was good enough to go on the night shift. The night shift is not like the day or the evening shift. The personnel are staffed to a minimum. You are down to two nurses and one orderly. That specific night, I was working with a nurse, Ms. Seals. She was blonde, stocky built and about 5'6" tall with a rather masculine demeanor. She spent five years in the military. This may explain why she behaved the way she did. One of the nurses called to be off that night. So, it was only Ms. Seals and me. They tried to get someone to come in, but the people who worked in the ER cherished their off days like they did their paychecks. Everyone knew that if you were called in, they were obviously short staffed. You would end up working like a Hebrew slave. So, no one came in.

For some strange reason, it wasn't busy that night. We only had the one patient with a history of drug addiction. They brought him in because he was shooting heroin into his left arm. The arm had become infected. It was twice the size of his right arm. This condition is called cellulitis. This patient was in excruciating pain.

This man was about 5'6" tall and approximately 190 pounds. He was very muscular with a lot of hair on his face and a very unkempt look. He kept asking me to give him something for pain. I told him that I was just an Orderly. I couldn't give him anything for pain, but I would tell the nurse. When I mentioned it to Ms. Seals, she informed me that she had just given him a pain shot. It would be another three to four hours before he could get anything else. I told the patient what she said. Then, 10 minutes later, he called me over to his bed. He said, "If you don't give me a pain shot, I'm going to do something bad to you." My reply was, "Look, I told you I'm just an Orderly. I don't give pain shots or any kind of shots. If you want a shot, you will have to take it up with the nurse or the doctor. He immediately leaped from the bed. He then pulled the front of my uniform, yanking me to the bed. Once he had me down, he started choking me. We wrestled to the ground. I was on top of Him, hitting him in the face but he had a firm hold on my throat. I knew Ms. Seals was going to call security. So, I tried to hold him off until security came. But to my surprise, she didn't call anyone. She was standing there cheering for me like this was a scheduled World Boxing Fight. In my mind I'm saying, "You fool, can't you see this man is killing me?" Well, I guess when I quit hitting him and fell to the ground, it was obvious that I wasn't winning. She knew once he got past me, she was next. Right away, she started pushing the buzzer for security. He started coming for her. She was pushing the buzzer and yelling, "Security, Security, come quickly!" Just as he grabbed her, they came in the door and made light work of him very quickly. Little did I know, this was just the beginning of many fights I would have in the ER.

There was a lot of crime in the city of Gary during that time. The street gangs were running rampant. They were killing so many people we were starting to lose count. I had my first encounter with the street gangs one evening when several of them came to the ER. This patient was taken to an isolated area in the city so they could assassinate him. He was about 6'2" tall and about 165 pounds. He wore a short Afro, neatly trimmed, and had a thick mustache.

This man was thin in appearance with a deep voice, but very neatly dressed. He wore nice silk slacks and a contrasting silk shirt.

He told me the gang was going to kill him because some of their money was missing. To spare his life, he showed them where he hid the money. While they were walking toward an old house in an abandoned area, he slugged one of the guys and made a break for the car. They started shooting at him. He was hit several times in the upper deltoid region of his right arm. Fortunately, he managed to get away. The injured man came straight to the ER. He drove his car right up to the door of the ER and jumped out. He ran down the hall yelling, "They are trying to kill me! They are trying to kill me! I've been shot!"

We were sitting at the nurse's station talking when we saw the man running up the hall, bleeding from the arm. So right away we put him on a bed to treat him. I went to the nurse's station to get the clipboard so we could write the patient up. The phone rang and I answered it. The voice on the other end said, "Do you have someone that just came in whose shot?" It was common for us to give out information on people being wounded. News traveled fast when someone was injured. Their family members and friends would call in to check on them. The guy asked, "Is he dead?" I said, "No, he is alive." Then he said, "Not for long," and hung up.

I went into the cubicle where the nurses and the doctors were and told them about the phone call. The man started screaming, "They are going to kill me! You got to hide me! I know too much! I know too much!" The staff became afraid and called security. Security never answered their page. We had no idea where they were. We knew there were times when they would leave the hospital to go get sandwiches. We never told anyone because they would look out for us too. Sometimes they would go to their girl-friend's houses. But whatever the reason was, they were nowhere to be found. The nurses were starting to pace. The doctor was sitting in a chair sweating. They were saying, "I'm not getting killed over some drug dealer." Since security is not here, we are leaving. The doctor said, "I'm leaving too." The only ones left were Ned and I. Ned had been there for a long time. He was the oldest Orderly we had. Ned was in his 50s and his head was starting to get bald. He was about 5'10" tall and approximately 240 pounds. He was fearless. He wasn't afraid of anyone. He had a stern look on his face as if he had everything under control. I liked working with Ned because he could really handle unruly people. The streets were the gang's turf, and the ER was Ned's turf. It was also rumored that Ned had a gun in his locker. I never saw it but I'm sure he did.

Ned said, "We will hide this guy in the cast room." This is the room the doctors take patients if they have bone fractures to get a cast applied. We decided to tell the gang that the guy was in surgery. Ned told the guy after we put him in the room, "You better not say a word." About 15 minutes later, we heard the shuffling sound of many feet as a crowd came closer to where we were. Approximately 50 young men came down the hall to the ER. They looked rough. Some had beards. Some had scars on their faces. Some had tattoos. Most of them had on black leather jackets with their caps turned backwards.

A gang member, obviously the leader, walked up to me and asked in a very serious, stern voice, "Where is he at?" He was short but stocky built. The man had a neatly trimmed beard on his rough, 30-year-old face. He was neatly dressed in his silk slacks and cowboy boots. His motorcycle jacket displayed an emblem of an Eagle on the front and back. I said, "Who are you talking about?" He said, "You know exactly who I'm talking about, the guy that got shot." Ned was in the office standing right behind me. I told the man that the guy was in surgery. He told his boys to check out all the rooms. The leader said, "Don't let me find out that you lied to me, or I will kill you!" I said, "Listen I can prove it to you!" I'm thinking fast now. My life depends on my response. I thought about the hospital emergency code.

The hospital had an emergency code that you could give the operator. If you gave her that code, she knew she was to immediately call the police. So, I called the operator and said, "Operator this is a code 10. Would you connect me to surgery?" She says, "Johnson, you know surgery is closed." I said, "Listen, I have people here in the ER that are looking for a gunshot victim and I need to verify it. So, I want you to expedite this to a code 10. She says, "Johnson, only the charge nurse can call a code 10." The gang member looked at me and said, "What did she say?" Ned looked at me and knew I was in deep trouble. He knew of a button that we had in the ER that would ring in the police station like a panic button. I never knew we had this button. So, Ned eased past me. He sat down in the chair and reached under the desk and pressed the button. The guy said, "Why are you stalling?" I said, "I'm not stalling. The operator doesn't seem to want to cooperate." Within minutes the police were on the ramp.

The policemen rushed in. When they saw this big gang of about 50 guys they immediately slowed down. The police passively walked by these men unaware of what is going on. They moved cautiously, watching their every move. There were about 10 policemen. The leader of the gang said, "So you called the police." I said, "No, I didn't call the police. You have been right here with me all the time. You know I didn't call the police."

Right at that time, the police officer spoke up. He said, "It doesn't matter who called us. All you guys can't be here in this emergency room. So, why are you here?" The leader of the gang said, "We were checking on one of our members that got shot."

25

That's when Ned spoke up and said, "We have been trying to tell these guys that the man is in surgery, but they don't want to leave." The officer then stated that they had to leave. The leader looked at me and said, "Don't let me find out that you are lying. I said, "Hey man, I have no reason to lie to you! I don't even know you!" He said in a low growl, "But I know you now and I won't forget your face." They left. I told Ned, "Man, if that wasn't close!"

I was so nervous. I was sweating so much that my shirt was soaking wet. Ned said, "Always remember this Johnson, never let them see you sweat. This is my emergency room. I run this." He said, "I just hate that I couldn't get to my locker to get my gun." I said, "Ned, maybe it's good you didn't. One gun doesn't stand a chance against 50." He said, "That's OK. If I got to go out, I'm going out smoking."

Then Ned said, "I bet everybody is in the coffee shop." So, he picked up the phone and called the coffee shop. Then he said, "You guys didn't have to leave," as he walked back and forth with the phone in his hand. He looked like a black super-hero that had just saved the day. "I had everything under control. You know when Big Ned is around; you don't have anything to worry about. I used to be a gang member too. I am not afraid of anybody. The police and me made them all leave. I probably could have put them out by myself, but it was so many I needed a little back up."

The staff came right back. The doctor said, "Where is the patient?" We told him that the patient was in the cast room. Doc had us to bandage the man up. None of his wounds were life threatening. Then Doc released him. The man begged us to keep him in the hospital and keep police protection around him. Doc said, "No, you brought this on yourself, and we are not going to risk everyone's life just to save yours."

The guy eased to the door, while looking outside to see if anyone was waiting for him. He noticed that the coast was clear. He ran down the ramp to his car and jumped in, taking off with the tires smoking. We never saw him again. Hundreds of patients are treated in the ER. Daily. It is impossible to monitor their status after their release.

The ER was non-stop action. I wish I could tell you about all the cases we saw. But I can only remember the ones that were colorful, funny, or emotionally draining. These events left an indelible impression on my mind. Even though these events happened years ago, I still find myself telling these stories.

One day, we were extremely busy. This man came running through the door. He was shouting that he had been shot in the hand. He was very handsome with dark curly hair and a nice thick mustache. He was dressed very neatly in a gold knit shirt with matching slacks. There was a young lady with him. She appeared to be in her 30s. She was about 5'7" tall and maybe 125 pounds. She was a very attractive woman. She was wearing a pair of Calvin Kline jeans with a brown cowboy shirt and boots.

One of the other medics picked up the patient's chart to write him up. We called him "Tricky Dick" because he thought he was so cool. Dick was cool. He was about 35 years old. He was a very well dressed, manicured man. His uniforms were always starched and pressed. Dick was single and always bragged about being the world's greatest player. Dick was about 5'9" tall and approximately 185 pounds with a medium-sized Afro haircut.

Dick took the man and put him on one of the beds. He yelled to me to bring him a clipboard.

When I went into the office to get one, the phone rang. I answered it. There was a lady's voice on the other end. She wanted to know if a man came in that had been shot in the hand. I said,

"Yes." She said, "I'm his wife. Would you please tell him I'm on my way up there now." She then hung up the phone. I went to the room and asked Dick to step out for a minute. I needed to have a word with him. I whispered and told him of the phone conversation. I asked him if we should tell the man? Obviously, the woman with him wasn't his wife. Dick said, "OH NO AND SPOIL THE SHOW! I told the head nurse, and she went to alert security. Dick went behind her and told security that we really didn't need them, we could handle it.

About 15 minutes later, a little short woman about 5'5" tall and looking to be in her mid-30s, and not weighing more than a 100 pounds entered the ER. Her short hair was styled very neatly. She had on a pair of nice polyester slacks and a nice linen top. The lady looked very concerned like most people do when they learn that their family members have been shot. She was a little out of breath, probably because she rushed to get to the hospital. She asked, "Which room is my husband in?" Dick said, "Who is your husband?" She said, "Mr. Banks." Dick said, "He is in cubicle number four." Dick looked at me and said, "It's show time!" We were laughing! I knew this wasn't right, so I stayed out of it.

Suddenly, we heard this yelling and cursing. Then the girlfriend came out from behind the curtain. She told the wife, "You wait right here! I'll be right back! I got somebody for you!" I said, "Dick she's going to get a gun!" He says, "I'm going to follow her. If she gets one, I'm going to take it from her." Then Dick came running back down the hall. He told me, "She went to get her sister! She went to get her sister!" He says, "Boy, little mama is going to have to fight now!" Up the hall came this big woman. She had very large arms and large breasts that flopped as she moved gracelessly down the hall. She was stomping and breathing hard like a big Brahma bull. She was about 6'1" tall and about 250 pounds with short hair. She looked like the kind of woman that would take no stuff. She said, "Where is she at! I'm going to teach her a lesson once and for all!" She went into the room and confronted the little woman. Suddenly, we heard this piercing scream! Then we saw the big woman run out of the cubicle with the little woman in her arms! The little woman had jumped into the big woman's arms and bit her right on the breast! That woman was running back and forth screaming and hollering! We were in the nurse's station trying to hold each other up. We were weak from laughing so hard. Even the other patients were bent over from laughter. She let the big woman go as she simultaneously hit her upside the head with her fist. That big woman turned, and down the hallway she ran! Then the little woman jumped on the girlfriend, and it wasn't long before she ran down the hallway too. And last, but not least, she jumped on her husband. He was taller and weighed much more than his wife. The sight of her coming after him made him run for it too! When she came out of the cubicle, everyone was cheering and saying, "Go head Little Sista; you know you bad!"

She walked down the hall like she had just won an Olympic gold medal in boxing. She held her head up high with a powerful stride and an extra dip in her walk. The look on her face said, I showed them! They all left the ER. We are not sure what happened to them after this event. I guess you are probably wondering why we let this happen. The ER can be stressful or monotonous. Due to the tension, the workers allow things to happen. These were welcomed moments.

CHAPTER 4

FEAR OF THE DEAD

SOME OF THE WORKERS IN THE HOSPITAL WOULD pull a lot of pranks. For instance, everyone knew about Donald Malcovich. He was an Orderly who had an uncanny fear of the dead. Donald was a nice guy, about 6'2" tall with blond hair, very thin and clumsy. He was in his early 20s and only weighed about 150 pounds. He was always falling over something. Donald would tell you that he wanted nothing to do with any one dead. At that time, it was routine for Orderlies to go to the morgue to get the morgue cart. They would return to the floor to put the dead person on it.

The morgue was in another section of the hospital. Once they delivered the corpse, the orderly tagged the toe, and the body was put in the cooler. On the day turn, all the Orderlies had to do was take the body to the morgue. The morgue attendant would do the rest. But on the evening and night shifts, you had to do it all.

All the nurses knew that Donald was afraid of dead people. They would only call him if there were no other males around to take the patient to the morgue. Most of the time they would call one of us in the ER and we would look out for Donald. But this specific day, we were just too busy. Donald was the only other Orderly on the floors.

The guys who worked in engineering were always playing jokes on Donald because they knew of his fear. The nurses told Donald to take the body down to the morgue and the attendant would take care of it. While Donald was waiting at the elevator, the guys in engineering saw him with the body so they decided to play a trick on him. They told him that he had been paged to come back to his floor. They offered to watch the body until he came back. So, while he was gone, they took the body to the morgue.

Setting up their little prank, they got another cart and put one of the engineers on it. They put a sheet over his face so Donald wouldn't notice. Unsuspectingly, Donald returned, not knowing the carts had been switched. He told the guys, "The nurses said they didn't call me." They said, "We thought we heard your name. We must have made a mistake. Would you like us to go with you and help you?" As scary as Donald was, you know he wasn't going to turn down the help. At that time, the morgue attendant had just left for lunch. When they arrived at the morgue, the guy on the cart started to raise up. He reached and grabbed Donald's hand. The hair on Donald's head stood straight up! He lost all the color in his face. He screamed like a woman in distress! He ran and jumped through a glass window! The engineers were all over the floor, rolling around laughing! All those guys got fired. They brought Donald to the ER. He had some cuts and scratches on his face and hands. After that incident he quit, and we never saw him again.

In the early 70s we didn't have ambulance services like we do today. The funeral home would provide ambulance services. They would pick up the sick and injured in a hearse and drive like maniacs to the hospital. The attendants didn't have to be medics. All they needed was some first aid training. There was one attendant whose name was Herman. Herman was a little short fat man who would steal the sweetening out of sugar. He was in his early

40s with gray in his hair and beard. Herman was about 5'6" tall with a potbelly. If Herman and his partner picked you up, you better try to stay conscious. Otherwise, you were subject to come to the ER with nothing on but your personality. Herman and his partner would roll those bodies. They took shoes, rings, coats, and hats, etc. It was not unusual for us to see Herman come into the ER with a hat too little for his head or rings too little for his fingers. The family would ask for the people's clothes, and we would say, "What clothes?" There were times when the patients would regain consciousness and ask for their shoes, coats, wallets and rings. When we informed them that they came in with nothing on, they would be furious. We would look at each other and say at the same time "Herman has struck again." Naturally, by this time he is long gone. The charge nurse would call the funeral home to inquire about the patient's personal belongings. But as expected, Herman knew nothing about the missing items.

Now the ER is starting to upgrade itself. All the guys in the ER had to go to school to become EMTs, (Emergency Medical Technicians) and they started a new procedure call triage. This is a procedure requiring the most urgent or critical patients be treated first. There was a desk and a cart in the lobby, so the EMT could critique or assess every patient that came in. The worst ones were sent straight to the ER. This new procedure was implemented to save more lives. It wasn't practical to leave someone in the lobby bleeding and take the patient back to be seen with a cold or fever because they came in first

Today it was my turn to work triage. As the patients would come in, I would write them up, take their vitals, and send the most urgent patients back first. This was one busy day. There were people everywhere. Some in chairs, some in wheelchairs, and people on crutches. They were carrying folks in that couldn't walk and needed a place to lie down. There also was no end to the injured kids and crying babies.

Suddenly, the doors opened and in came Herman. He had a man on his cart that had been shot through the eye. I sent him straight back to the ER. Herman told the doctor he thought the man was dead. At that time, if the doctors were very busy, it wasn't unusual for some of them to take one look at the patient and if he looked dead, pronounce him dead. Then they would send them to the morgue. Normally, if the doctors weren't busy, they would check the patient for vital signs, and if there were no vital signs, they would pronounce him dead.

Most of the time when they pronounced a person dead, they would be right. This time was different. The bullet went through the man's eye and came out his temple. On the way out, it must have concussed the skull to render the man unconscious (to concuss means to shake up or cause injury to). The fact that he had lost so much blood attributed to his breathing being extremely shallow. We also must factor in he was brought in by Herman. He probably spent more time checking the patient for valuables than checking the patient.

The ER doctor was from India. He was a small man about 130 pounds, in his middle 30s and about 5'6" tall. He was new to the ER and would get very nervous when a lot of trauma patients came in. More than once, I witnessed him pronouncing a patient dead without checking to see if he was dead. This guy looked dead. He had blood all over his face.

The hospital had moved the morgue from the opposite end of the hospital closer to the ER since so many people were being brought in DOA (or Dead-on Arrival). In fact, the door to the morgue was right in the lobby next to triage. There was a big sign on the door that said MORGUE. The people in the lobby saw

Herman take the body to the morgue. They also saw the morgue attendant leave for the day. The morgue attendant had put the man in the cooler. About a half an hour later the man regained consciousness. He said he felt cold, and he couldn't see anything. It was pitch dark. Then he felt his face and noticed his eye was gone. He started to feel around the cooler, and he only felt the cold metal walls. He noticed, as he started moving, whatever he was laying on would roll. So, he kept pushing until the slab rolled all the way out. Then he climbed out of the cooler. The room was dark because the attendant had shut the lights off. He started feeling his way around the walls. Once he felt the doorknob, he tried to open the door, but his hands had so much blood on them they kept slipping off. So, he knocked on the door.

Picture this! Everyone knows that the only people that go into the morgue are dead people. They also saw everyone leave. So, who in the world would be knocking on the door from the inside? When he knocked the first time, all eyes focused on the door. He knocked again. Now everyone is starting to sit up. People are starting to get a little antsy. I must confess I'm getting nervous too. He knocked one more time. A man sitting close to the door got up and went over and opened the door. In the doorway stood a man about 6'0" tall in a hospital gown. There was blood all over his face and all over the gown. Looking at his face, there was one eye and a hole where the other eye should be. He was just standing there. The people in the lobby froze. The man said, "Where am I?" Everything with feet started to run! People ran off and left their babies. People got out of their wheelchairs and started running. The people that were carried in that said they couldn't walk jumped up off the carts and ran, obviously in fear. The man walked toward me and said, "Why is everybody running?" Now it's time for me to go! I ran outside and came around to the back door of the ER to tell everybody about the dead man that walked out of the morgue. Before I could say anything, the man was coming down the hall toward the ER.

The Indian doctor had just walked out of the doctor's room and looked the dead man right in his face. He immediately fell to his knees and started praying in his native tongue. The nurses and all the patients cleared the ER. People who had seen Herman bring the man in were screaming, "That is the dead man! That is the dead man!" as they were running. The man was getting frustrated now and said, "Why is everybody running? I am not going to hurt you!" Then he walked over to the doctor who was still down on his knees praying and said, "Hey doc will you please tell me what is going on? Am I hurt that bad?"

The doctor slowly but carefully tried to get up. It was obvious he was scared out of his wits. He gathered himself as he rose to his feet. He looked the man in the face and tried to speak. He was shaking so bad he had trouble getting his words out. He said, "I pronounced you dead! You were shot in the head right through the eye!" The patient said, "Look at me Doc. Do I look like I am dead? I know I am a bloody mess, but I am not dead!"

I saw the doctor and the man talking. So, I slowly started going toward them. The doctor saw me and said, "Johnson, tell everyone to come back because this man is not dead. We need to treat him right away." So, slowly everyone started to come back in. My heart was really beating fast just from the thought of what we had seen. Some of the nurses were still a little afraid to come near this man. A lot of the patients left and did not come back. I guess the excitement was a little bit too much for one day.

The doctor examined the man and declared him a medical miracle. The probability of someone sustaining an injury of that nature and surviving is very remote. Their only hypothesis of how the bullet missed the brain was that it hit a bone in the orbit and was deflected coming out of the temporal area. You can call it luck, fate, or just plain being blessed, but this man walked away from death. They admitted him to the hospital and operated on his eye. He remained there for several weeks, and then he was released. I have heard of people getting shot point-blank in the head and getting up and walking away. This time I had the opportunity to be an eyewitness to it.

CHAPTER 5

CODE SEVEN

IN THE ER, THERE ARE SO MANY THINGS GOING on that you never know what to expect next. You get to see people with mental problems that go above and beyond what is normal. One afternoon while we were busy working on a lot of colds and fevers, three huge men looking like they could be NFL linebackers came up the hallway dragging a little short man. His name was Andre. They had his hands tied with chicken wire. So obviously our first thought was why would these huge men need to tie this little man up in chicken wire just to bring him in? But in a few moments, it became as clear as day why they needed that type of restraint. This little guy appeared to be about 5'5" or 5'6" tall and probably not a 100 pounds soaking wet. He was probably 28 or 29 years old. He was throwing these men around like pieces of tissue paper.

The doctor, ascertaining that they had a serious problem on their hands, told us to put him in the Psych room (this is the room where we place mental patients). We were to restrain him immediately. Even with his hands tied with the chicken wire he still fought, giving these guys all they could handle. As a matter of fact, they were not handling him. Instead, he was manhandling them. The bed was already setup with four-point flannel restraints. This made it possible to restrain his hands and feet.

We got him in the bed and restrained his hands and feet. He broke the flannel like you would pop a piece of string. We ran and got the leather restraints. We had to wrestle him down with the three big guys sitting on him. After we got the leathers applied to his hands and feet, we felt secure. As we turned to walk away, we heard a loud snap. We didn't want to believe what we saw as we turned and looked back at the little man. Never, since I've been in the ER, has a man of his size broken leather restraints.

He snapped his hands free like you would break a cracker; it was nothing! Once his hands were free, he tried to break his feet free. This is when we all grabbed him. We had to get security to come down and physically handcuff his hands to the bed.

The doctor told the nurse to give him a shot to help calm him down. We sighed with relief. The three big men who brought him in said he set the house on fire and went outside and turned a car over on its hood. Had we not seen this display of his strength, there is no way we would have believed their story just looking at this man. Amazingly, an hour after the shot was given, he was as gentle as a lamb. He was calm and docile while the doctor examined him. The doctor felt it was safe for us to take him out of restraints. The little man assured us that he was fine now. We called his family, and they came to pick him up.

One week later, I was on the 3 p.m.-to-11 p.m. shift. We heard a noise that sounded like someone had just knocked the whole door in. Frank and I jumped up and ran out of the nurse's station to see what was going on. Frank was another EMT hired to work in the ER. Several of the EMTs working for the Gary Fire Department had acquired second jobs working in the ER. Dick was hired this way too. The two of us noticed the three big men were back, dragging this little guy in again. I said, "Oh no, not him again!" The staff on duty at that time was unaware of his magnificent feats of strength, but I was. The three big men had the chicken wire tied so tight around his wrists that they were bleeding from him trying to break free.

I immediately called security because I knew the restraints weren't going to hold him. We had to take wire cutters to get the chicken wire off his hands. I informed the doctor of his prior visit and the kind of strength he exhibited when he came in the first time. The doctor decided to admit him, especially after the three big men told us he had broken all the furniture in his house. The doctor had the nurse give him a shot to help calm him down once again. After he calmed down, they admitted him to a medical floor.

I happened to be the one to take him to the floor. I took security with me just as a precaution. He kept assuring us that he was OK and that he would not try to harm anyone. After the nurses read his chart, they wanted him secured in flannel restraints. He really didn't want the restraints, but we did it anyway. He protested but to no avail. I had just left the unit and as I was about to get on the elevator to go back to the ER, I heard over the loudspeaker, "CODE SEVEN, CODE SEVEN! TWO EAST!" I knew it had to be "Little Man."

CODE SEVEN was a special signal the hospital had devised to get as much manpower to the scene as possible. Anytime they called CODE SEVEN, every male in the house had to go to the designated area. Most of the time it was a situation where you would need a lot of men to restrain someone. I ran back around the corner. Just as I thought, the little man had broken his hands free and was working on his feet. The nurses were terrified and called CODE SEVEN. We immediately grabbed him and tried to hold him down. Four large security officers came in and told us to move, and that they would get him. Two of them were on his right and the other two were on his left. He literally picked them up off their feet. One of the officers said, "I weigh 250 pounds. This little guy picked me up like it was nothing! Where is he getting his strength from?" It wasn't until the nurses gave him a shot that they were able to get him restrained.

The next day, I had just taken a patient to the floor he was on. I noticed him walking toward the nurse's station. One of the guys in security happened to be sitting there talking to one of the nurses. When he came near me, I asked him, "Andre, where are you going?" He said, "I'm going down to the cafeteria to get something to eat." I told him, "They don't let the patients leave the floor." Then I asked him, "Weren't you in restraints?" He said, "Yeah, but I broke those easily."

The nurse jumped up and said, "Andre, go back to your room right now!" The security got up and walked up to Andre and said, "The nurse said you have to go back to your room." This guy was a slim blond-haired, medium-build man about 6'0" tall with a real cocky attitude. I pulled him gently by the arm and whispered in his ear, "You are going to need some backup. This man has the strength of 10 men. He obviously was unfamiliar with Andre because his reply was, "I don't need any backup to put this little man back in bed." Andre said, "Don't walk up on me. And I'm not going back to bed!" I said, "Oh no, this is going to get ugly!" I whispered to the nurse, "Call CODE SEVEN. Call CODE SEVEN!" Andre grabbed his gown by the neck and ripped it in half. When the officer grabbed Andre, he grabbed the officer by the collar and under his legs. Then he quickly hoisted him into the air while throwing him into the window! Fortunately, the window was closed. He rolled off the window and down to the floor. Either he was dazed, or he was just afraid to get up. Either way, he laid there. I started to notice something about Andre. The only time he gets this surge of strength is when he gets angry or agitated. The nurses started screaming! Andre looked like the hero of the day. He walked away casually on his way to the cafeteria. There was no way I was going to get in his way.

You could hear CODE SEVEN ringing all over the loud-speaker. Suddenly men came from everywhere. They grabbed Andre and one by one he threw them off him. They eventually got him down but with much difficulty. After they got him down, I jumped in to assist. The officers handcuffed him and physically drug him back to his bed. The nurse then gave him something to settle him down.

An entire week had gone by, and I was surprised we hadn't had a CODE SEVEN on Andre. I thought maybe he had been released to go home. We had a patient who was admitted to that floor from the ER. They asked me to take her up to her room. I put the lady in the bed and walked out to the nurse's station to talk to one of the nurses. She was sitting in the chair at the desk, and I was sitting on the desk looking down at her. I asked her if Andre had been discharged? She said, "No, but he has been acting very civil." Suddenly, I see these three nurses running toward me screaming, "Y'all better run! Y'all better run!"

The three nurses were trying to fix Andre's bed without taking him out of restraints. Andre became agitated. He broke the restraints, and he broke part of the wooden rail off the headboard. One nurse was so terrified, because he was between her and the door. The other two nurses were by the door, able to exit the room. They told her, "We are going to try to distract him. When we do, leap over the bed, and run for your life." The trapped nurse was not young, nor was she small. She was in her 50s and full figured. But don't let anybody tell you a person can't move when they're scared. The two nurses ran to the head of the bed. When he swung at them, that cleared the way for her to run. She leaped over that bed like an Olympic track star and down the hall they came. If you are wondering what I did at this point, stop wondering. Here are three nurses running toward me. Andre is behind them with a big stick in his hand. He has nothing on but a hospital gown that is blowing in the wind. Now tell me what would you do? Exactly.

The nurses and I all took off running. Down the stairs we went. Everyone we ran into received the same message. "You better run! You better run!" He chased us from the second floor to the first floor. The crowd that is running is starting to get bigger. No one had time to stop and call CODE SEVEN. To do so, you would have to stop and deal with Andre.

We ran out the door and on to the street. Finally, security ran out and tackled Andre on the grass. Andre is in rare form today! While he is throwing policemen down, his gown is up around his neck. The whole world can see what God gave him. But Andre was too busy to care. Someone must have called CODE SEVEN because all the men in the house started to come out and got into the wrestling match. I would have lent them a hand, but I was too exhausted. After about 15 minutes of Andre putting on a show and a darn good one, I might add, they finally got him down.

People had stopped their cars. Everyone in the area came over to watch the show. They hand cuffed him and drug him back into the hospital. Right away, they gave him another shot to calm him down. The next day they took Andre to surgery and took something out of his brain. We never knew exactly what happened, but he was soon released from the hospital, and we never saw him again.

That was not the end of CODE SEVEN.

We got a call to come to the Psych Unit. That day, I was working with my good friend Dick. As usual, he was cool, neat as a pin and not afraid of anybody. Dick was a little older than me so I looked up to him. Dick said, "Come on Johnson, let's go up here and handle this situation." When we got to the fourth floor, we noticed all the guys standing outside the door of the Psych Unit. Dick said swaggeringly, "What's the problem?" The guys said go inside and you'll see. So, Dick said, "Stand aside and let some real men go in. Come on Johnson." We walked in the door. Dick asked the nurse, "What's the problem?" She said, "We have a patient in the next room that doesn't want to take his shot." Dick said, "He's going to take his shot." When we walked to the room, the man stood up. As he stood, I thought I'd never see the end of him. This man was tall! He was dark skinned with a baldhead. He had muscles where Dick and I didn't have meat. He looked at Dick and me and said, "You going to give me a shot? I want to see you try it." Dick looked at me. He looked at the nurse. As he was walking backwards, he said, "You're right, you don't have to have a shot tonight." The guy said, "That's what I thought as he sat back down." But in the door came my real hero, Eddie.

Eddie was a policeman. Not just an ordinary policeman. He was one of the most feared guys in the hospital. He didn't take any stuff from anyone. I do mean no one. He was so mean that when most people would see him coming, they would get in line. Eddie was about 6'2" tall and he also had a baldhead. He was very muscular with a mean Terminator look. He commanded so much respect. As he walked up the hallway approaching the door, the guys started cheering. Eddie really gets this macho look on his face as if Superman has just arrived. As he moved down the hall toward the room, the guys parted to let him through like Moses parted the Red Sea. He walks in the door and says, "What's the problem?" Dick and I looked at each other and said, "That guy is going to get it now." The nurse told Eddie that the man wouldn't take his shot. Eddie said, "Where is he at?" We all pointed to the room. Eddie walked up to the room. This big dark

45

man stood straight up. He said, "You going to give me this shot? I want to see you try it." Eddie looked the guy up and down, sizing him up. Then he looked at us and the nurse and said, "If the man doesn't want a shot, he doesn't have to have one." He turned and left. I asked Eddie why he didn't make the guy take a shot. His reply was, "There are some people even bullets won't hurt. Only a fool would tackle a man that big, and crazy too!" So obviously sometimes the patients do win out.

There was a time when they would call CODE SEVEN and I would run like Carl Lewis to get to the destination. But, after you have been to a few, you learn not to walk so fast. In fact, I would just walk up slowly, hoping the problem has been resolved before I get there.

We say a lot about the men, but the women were just as bad. They called CODE SEVEN for the third floor, Room 350. When we got there the nurses looked like they had been through World War III. Their clothes had been ripped and their hair was all over their heads. In the middle of the floor stood a little woman. She was 4 x 4 x 4. She didn't want to go to bed. She stated this emphatically, "And no one is going to make me!" I walked up to her and said, "Miss, you are going to have to go to bed." She hit me with a backhand so hard, I fell backwards and skidded under the desk. At first, I was shocked. This was the hardest lick I had ever had! She started slinging guys and throwing them like she was a professional wrestler. After a few minutes, we stopped to collect ourselves and assess the damages. We couldn't do anything with that little woman!

She looked at us and saw one of the guys in the crowd that she liked. She grabbed him and said, "You going to make love to me!" She ripped his shirt completely off his back. She threw him to the ground and jumped on top of him. He was hollering and screaming like a little girl saying, "Get her off me! Get Her off me!" Most men fantasize about occasions like this. But obviously, this wasn't such an occasion. We finally got her off this guy and got her back to bed. As we left the room she says, "Thanks boys, can we play like this again tomorrow?"

There were many other CODE SEVENS over the years. The hospital instituted another program for dealing with these kinds of problems. I can honestly say handling CODE SEVEN situations proved to be some of the most challenging.

CHAPTER 6

HOW I BECAME A PARAMEDIC

Two years have passed since I began working in the ER. When I first started there, I was as green as an apple. Now I am considered an old pro. The hospital decided to upgrade their emergency room to the same status as those hospitals in Illinois. The Illinois hospitals had instituted a new procedure. It was the EMT Program. This is the Emergency Medical Technicians. They decided that giving basic life support in the field would help save more lives. They were also getting away from the old funeral home service of rendering first aid. No longer would you see a hearse responding to emergencies. Now you will see the wiener-style ambulances that are manned by certified EMTs. Most of the cities decided to let their fire department personnel become EMTs. Dick and all the other guys that worked for the fire department and worked in the ER were sent to EMT school.

The fire department would be responsible for maintaining the ambulance and its personnel. Lutheran General Hospital had just hired the director of the EMT Program from Illinois. They wanted to upgrade the emergency room. So, he was put in charge of emergency services. As Orderlies, we were told that we would have to go back to school. We had to become EMTs to maintain our jobs in the ER. They also appointed one of the nurses to assist the director in the new training program. Her job was to make sure all the male Orderlies were properly trained.

The first wave of guys went through. The training took three months. All the guys passed. I didn't get in the first wave because the class was full. She later told me not to worry, that I would be in the second wave. One of the suburban cities was trying to get their EMTs trained so they could start their ambulance service. Unfortunately, they only had a month before the deadline to get the ambulance service started. The hospital started a special accelerated class to get these guys certified. My nurse director told my buddy, Sam, and me since we were the last two waiting to get certified, she had decided to put us in the accelerated class. She said, "I know it might be a little fast-paced for you, but you guys seem to catch on fast. I'm convinced you can handle it."

This nurse was not particularly fond of Sam or me. She was slyly trying to put us in a position to be removed from the ER by putting us in this class. Her insincere confidence in us was punctuated by our knowledge of how she really felt. She just couldn't adjust to the style and confidence that we had in the ER. She didn't have to hold our hands or tell us what to do. We simply knew our jobs well.

Sam and I both felt that the class would be too fast paced for us, so we told her this. She said, "These guys who need to get certified have strong medical backgrounds like you and Sam. Some have been hospital core-men in the military. Also, several of the guys were in college for pre-med. You guys have been around for a few years, that is why I put you there." Sam said, "If we don't pass, we lose our jobs." She says, "Oh, you are going to pass, I've got confidence in you." If you could just see behind the fake smile and the façade of support and concern, you would know she was thirsting for our failure.

The class started. The pace was crazy! We barely had time to do the reading. A week passed, and Sam is starting to show signs of weakness. He came to me and said, "Johnson, I'm not going to make it." I said, "What do you mean, Sam?" He said, "They are going too fast, I can't keep up." I said, "Sam, please don't give up, I'll help you! We have got to stick together! If you quit, you are giving her just what she wants!" I really felt bad for Sam because he loved the ER. He was so good. He was the reason I was there. After doing everything possible to get me there, he then taught me everything about the ER. He greeted all the patients with a smile and all the doctors liked him. He was an asset to the ER.

We had only been in the class for about a week and a half when Sam came to me and said, "I can't digest this stuff that fast, and I'm going to have to cash it in." It really hurt me to see my buddy lose his job. She could have put Sam in a longer class, but she wanted Sam out. I made a commitment to myself right then. Whatever it took, I was going to pass this class. I was going to do it for me. I was going to do it for Sam. I was going to do it for all the brothers that were trapped in a similar way by the kind of hate that has permeated this society.

I reflected on the guys in Vietnam who were probably being overrun by the Viet Cong. What were they going to do for survival? They did what they were trained to do in a time of crisis. They had to dig in and put up a strong defense. I was of the same mindset. I was going to survive. So, I dug in. I studied like a man possessed, even though I had to do a full day's work at the hospital and endure the full load of the class. I was exhausted but relieved because at the end of the month, I passed my finals and qualified to take the Certification test. Yes! I passed my test! Now I'm a certified, bonafide, and stamped on both sides, EMT.

I wore my patch proudly. I stood with my head high. There was confidence in my walk and a smirk on my face, thinking, you thought you got me but I'm still here.

The doctors were starting to put more confidence in Dick and me since we qualified as EMTs. They felt that Dick and me showed promise of one day becoming physicians. Under their close supervision, we were taught how to suture. This is putting stitches in a wound. We got a lot of practice during the midnight shift. The ER took on its usual life. People were walking in, running in or being drug in. The ambulances were up and flying! They kept us busy! The doctor needed a lot of help and good help. So, the training they gave Dick and I really paid off. The ER had good medics and good nurses but only two good doctors. The rest were, "Just Doctors."

We were taught well by the good doctors. They showed us how to put casts on arms and legs. They also showed us how to do cut-downs (this is when a person has no visible veins, and you must make an incision in the skin to find a vein for starting an IV). We were also taught how to assist putting in chest tubes. These are tubes that are put through the rib cage into the lungs. This is used when a person's lung has collapsed. We learned how to manage gunshot wounds to the chest and the abdomen and how to manage all kinds of major fractures from car accidents, falls, etc. We still had to factor in the drunks we had to fight, the mental cases we ran from, and the regulars who always complained. "Why am I waiting so long"? "When is my turn?" "Are there any doctors working tonight?"

When "Just Doctors" worked, they would lean on Dick and me a lot. They knew of our dedication to doing a good job and of the training we had received. They would call our names all night long. But I loved it! It made me feel that I was worth my weight in gold. I was saving lives. I was on the cutting edge. I was as close to being a doctor as I could get at that time.

Dick was his usual cocky self. They say that knowledge can be a dangerous thing in the hands of certain people. Dick would let everyone know when he or she was less qualified than him. If the doctors did a procedure wrong, Dick would call them out on it. If the medics and nurses were slacking, Dick would rip into them like a staff sergeant did his troops. I can hear him now. "We are here to save lives. If you don't want to work, go home!" Dick was intimidating at times. When "Just Doctors" worked, they would confer with him first before treating certain patients.

Dick was very sensitive to how the elderly were treated. He always said he wanted to treat them like he would treat his parents. Even though the patient wasn't his parent, they were somebody's parent. One of the doctors asked Dick before he discharged an elderly man to look at the man and tell him what he thought. The man had been drinking and most of the time these people were released quickly. But Dick was on duty that night, and everyone was going to get treated right. Dick asked the doctor what kind of tests were run on the man? The doctor said, "I didn't run any. The man is just drunk." Dick said, "Doc, I drink too. But, if I ever come in here sick and you smell alcohol on my breath and just send me home without checking me out thoroughly, I'm going to have your job. Most of the elderly people I know feel that if you don't feel good, one good drink should straighten it out." The man was admitted to the hospital for acute pancreatitis. If Dick had not worked that night, the man might have died. Yes, Dick was arrogant, and he thought he was God's gift to medicine, but he was good for the patients coming to the ER.

Some of the doctors were interesting characters. One such character was Dr. Sykes. He was a tall man, and slim with long arms and blond hair. He was arrogant. He had a mean scowl that made people not want to get near him. Maybe he did it to make sure they stayed away. He had a year-round suntan. He was a hunter. He went to Africa at least three times a year. Each time he came back from his hunting expedition, he would come to the ER with something to show that he had been hunting. He had a cap and boots made from animals he killed. He was obviously a better hunter than he was a doctor. Dr. Sykes had no people skills and very poor bedside manner. He disliked ethnic people. He hated to treat the poor and underprivileged. He was a very wealthy man and he didn't mind letting you know it. He was a poster child for "Just Doctors."

One cold winter morning, the ambulance doors burst open. The medics were screaming, "We got a gunshot wound to the abdomen! It's a kid. He's only 10 years old!" We jumped straight up and rushed the patient into the trauma room. When we pulled the covers back to examine the wound, we noticed a wound the size of a big mush ball right in the center of his abdomen. The child's face was pale. He had a terrified look on his face with tears running from his eyes. He was a thin child, tall for his age. As he lay there moaning in pain, we worked frantically, trying to save this child's life.

Children always bring out the team's best in trauma situations. The doctors, the nurses and the staff know they must use their skills as quickly and judiciously as possible. They are painfully aware that time is of the essence. There is no greater joy than to give a child back to their parent. There is also no greater pain than to tell a parent that you couldn't save their child.

We jumped right in! Putting pressure bandages on the wound to try to control the bleeding. The nurses were busy trying to start an IV. I put an oxygen mask on the young man. This is routine for anyone that is bleeding because they become oxygen deficient as they lose blood.

Dr. Sykes was trying to clamp off some bleeders. The child pulled back the oxygen mask and asked him, pleading in a weak frightened voice, "Doctor, am I going to die?" The reply of this unfeeling, coldhearted doctor haunts me to this day. He looked at the child with a very nervous, unsure expression on his face. He opened his mouth and said, "Of course you are going to die! Do you think I can save you with a hole in your stomach this big?" The child took a long look at Dr. Sykes and laid back on the bed. His eyes rolled back in his head, and he never said anything after that. He closed his eyes and died right there in front of us.

The medics knew from previous experiences with Dr. Sykes that he was not a good trauma doctor. Trauma patients made him very nervous because all the pressure was on him, and he really wasn't sure of himself. His trauma skills were very poor. We were working frantically trying to keep this child alive until the trauma team arrived because we knew that if we left it up to Dr. Sykes, we might as well call a priest. Dr. Sykes gave this child no hope; not even an inch of willpower to hold on to life. In severe trauma cases we pull out all the stops because Dr. Sykes, "Just Doctor," wasn't going to pull any. He wasn't going to offer any encouragement.

The will to live is the strongest will of man. I have seen people hurt worse. The words, "Just hang in there, we are going to save you, don't give up," has had amazing effects on people in life-threatening situations.

Our Charge Nurse, Marlene, reached across the table, grabbing Dr. Sykes by the collar. She said, "I should kill you! Why would you tell a patient something like that! You gave that child no hope whatsoever!" Dr. Sykes said, "Hey, I didn't shoot the kid!

I'm not the babysitter! If these kids go out and get themselves shot and killed don't blame me! I'm not Jesus! I can't save them!"

Marlene was a full-figured, African American nurse. She was a very good trauma nurse. It took us a few minutes to pull Marlene off Dr. Sykes. When she let him go, his hair was all over his head and he was as red as a beet. She choked him good! The only reason we pulled Marlene off the doctor was because we didn't want her to lose her job. She did what we were feeling should have been done. That is why we didn't react right away to rescue him. He got what he deserved.

We separated the two. Marlene said, "I'm ok, let me go!" She adjusted her uniform, patted her hair back down and turned to face Dr. Sykes with a very angry, stern look. She shouted in a very firm voice, "I'm writing you up! I'm going to make sure we get you out of this emergency room!" Dr. Sykes went to go to the doctor's room to get composed. He turns and says to her in his arrogance, "I don't care who you tell! I have enough money to buy this place! You will be the one looking for a job!"

Things didn't go so well for Dr. Sykes after that. He was in love with a little Swedish nurse that worked in the ER. She was blonde and beautiful. She had sparkling hazel eyes. Her personality was as warm as her beauty. Everyone loved her Swedish accent. She was loved so much that almost every man in the hospital wanted to date her. It was rumored that half of them did. Dr Sykes found out and did he hit the ceiling! He looked at me and said, "What are you laughing at?" I said, "I know you didn't think you were the only man that she wanted." He told me, "You had better be glad you aren't in Africa. If so, I would hunt you." I told him, "You hunt things that can't hunt back." I looked at him thinking, hunting me might be dangerous for you. I said, "Don't let the hunter get captured by the game."

A week later, Dr. Sykes went back to Africa on a hunting expedition. When he arrived back home, he died. They say he contracted a rare disease while in Africa. As much as I didn't like this person, I still felt I was taught to have great regard for human life. The day we heard that he died, we got some money together to send flowers to the family. His wife told us he was already buried. She buried him the very next day. As cold as he treated others, that is how he was treated at death. Maybe she buried him quickly because of the disease that caused his death. Or, maybe he was as cold to her as he was to the patients.

When "Just Doctors" need medical attention, do they get what they gave to others? If that's the case, then Dr. Sykes got what he deserved again.

I encountered, and worked with, a lot of interesting people in the emergency room. But, after two years, the routine was starting to bore me. I didn't know what I was looking for, but I needed something to stimulate my interest. At that time my wish was granted. As EMTs, we were made aware that a new program was about to be implemented. It was the paramedic program. Anyone that had been an EMT for more than a year and had a sponsoring hospital, or ambulance service, qualified to get into the program. The program required one year of training. The training included learning basic and advanced life support. We would also receive clinical time in the hospital in surgery to learn how to intubate. We would spend time in the lab learning how to draw blood. We would spend time with the IV team learning how to start IVs. We also had to log 100 hours of supervised paramedic runs.

I signed up right away. The course proved to be very difficult. We started out with 40 students. Only 16 graduated. We lost half of the students in the first module. We had to learn things like acid base balance, anatomy, physiology, and pharmacology. We also had to learn a protocol for every emergency that you would encounter in the field. This protocol taught us how to treat the emergency with basic and advanced life support.

My two-year civilian duty time was up. I could return to the mills. After returning to my old job, I found it very difficult to keep up with the pace of the paramedic's class. They allowed me to work straight midnights so that I could go to school. I worked at the hospital in the evenings and went to school during the day. I had no free time to study. I had no time to rest. I slept on the job and between jobs. I was a walking Zombie.

I went to the Director of ER and asked her if she could put me on part-time. She informed me that they didn't have any part-time shifts available. She says, "If you can't keep up, maybe you need to drop the class and take it at another time." I was not going to drop the class. It was about my pride. Before we started the paramedic's course, one of the Charge Nurses, Laura, and I were involved in a heated discussion because Dr. Mesta wanted me to assist him in a full arrest on one of the floors. Any time they called full arrest, the ER doctors had to go to the patient's room to run the code. As I was leaving with Dr. Mesta, Laura asked, "Where are you going?" My reply was, "I'm going to assist Dr. Mesta." She says, "They don't need you. There is nothing you can do." I said, "That's not true. I can do CPR. I can be a runner; there is a lot I can do." Her reply was, "They need people up there that know what they are doing. They don't need any dummies." I said, "That's ok, I'll be in paramedic's school next week and when I finish, I want you to call me a dummy then." This was another reason I couldn't give up.

I really needed to be on part-time in the ER. If I expected to pass this class, I had to free up some more study time. Drastic times call for drastic measures. I decided to talk to the Assistant Vice-President over the ER. I asked him if there were any part-time positions available. He said, "Yes there are." I went back to my director and told her what the Assistant V.P. said. The look on her face was worth a million dollars. The color dropped from her face. Her mouth fell wide open. For a few seconds she was speechless. She said, "Well, let me go talk to him. Maybe things have changed, and I haven't been made aware of it."

By the way, she and Laura were good friends. You know, the nurse who called me stupid. Obviously, they were working together. I'm sure she never thought I would go over her head. When she came back, she said "I've got great news for you. I have convinced him to give you part-time. As she stood there with that fake smile, these questions went through my head. Why didn't she give me part-time when I first asked for it? Why did I have to go over her head? Why does she now want me to think she is doing me a big favor? I didn't say anything. I just thanked her and left. She probably still thinks that she conned me, but it doesn't matter. All I wanted was a schedule change. I didn't know that my paramedic instructor was a friend of my director and of Laura's.

Now it's all coming back to me. I recall my first day in the paramedic's class. My instructor approached me saying, "I've heard about you trying to play doctor in the emergency room. I'm letting you know right now that I'm going to be watching you very closely. If you do anything I don't like, you are out of this program." I didn't know why she singled me out like that. But as things started to unfold, it all started to make sense.

Class took off with a bang. We were really learning a lot. The course study was very difficult. If you couldn't keep up, you were just lost. I was struggling and barely hanging on.

The first module had just ended. You had to have a 77% average to stay in the program. I had a 77% average. My instructor approached me again and said, "Johnson, the second module is harder than the first. My suggestion to you at this time, since you are barely passing, is to get out and take it at another time. Unless you work a miracle, I don't see how you are going to make it."

I knew I had to make some drastic changes. My shift manager in the mill was upset with me because I was given the straight midnight shift to go to school. He had changed my schedule several times, putting me on the day shift. I, in turn, went to his manager and explained to him what I was trying to do. I said, "If I were allowed to finish school, I would be an asset to the Mill Personnel. There would be someone on staff trained in emergency medicine." He agreed and overruled my shift manager.

To punish me, my shift manager put me on the worst job they had at night. I went back to his manager and made him aware of how I was being treated. He assured me that he would take care of it. They assigned me to jobs that weren't so hectic. I figured with my new setup I would have more time to study, and I could work this miracle that my paramedic instructor said I would need.

I went to her office and told her that I would make a deal with her. I stated, "Allow me to stay in the class until midterm. If my grades haven't improved, I will resign." To my surprise, she accepted. I'm sure in her mind she thought I was not going to make it.

The second module started with us learning how to read EKGs (electrocardiogram). This is a reading of the heart rhythm. We had to learn what is normal and what is abnormal. I took to EKGs like a fish to water. I've always wanted to learn how to read them after watching doctors read them in the emergency room. Since my job wasn't so hectic at night, I would take my protocol and study it backwards and forwards. I would take out a pad and try to write each code from memory. For example: Code One – The first thing you do is your assessments. Then you take vitals. Give the patient oxygen. Put them in a comfortable position to breath. Dress all wounds, etc.

My grades had improved. I was averaging between 96%–98%. You would think my instructor would have offered encouragement by saying, "You have surprised me. You have done a good job. Keep up the good work." No............. She was still very hard on me. She would call on me constantly to answer a question and I dare not get it wrong. She would say, "This is what I'm talking about. Some of you think because you are carrying high averages you are going to pass this class. But I have news for you. I don't care if your average is 190%. If I don't think you can do this work, I'm not going to pass you." When she said that, she looked right at me. Can you imagine how that made me feel?

I knew right then things were going to be rough. But I said to myself, "I'm not giving up. Whatever I have to do, I will do. But I'm not giving up."

After six months of intensive training, I learned that the most important thing for a paramedic to know is the protocol. This is a list of how to treat all the emergencies in the field. I knew that I had to be able to recite it in my sleep if I planned to pass her class. I studied it over and over again. When I went to work at night in the Steel Mill, I would take a section of the protocol, study it, and then try to write as much as I could from memory. The job that they put me on was operating a front-end payloader or a bulldozer. I was either loading trucks or pushing ore. When I finished, or was on my break, I would try to get in as much studying as I could.

Working at night presented challenges indeed. Most of the time, the only light I had on the equipment I was running would be a flashlight. The only other source of light was a pen I borrowed from the hospital ER. I would hold the pen light in my mouth so I could see what I was writing. Then, I would position my flashlight to the right side of my protocol journal so I could see it. As difficult as it was to learn under these circumstances, I soon learned the protocol. It was such a good feeling to know that I had succeeded in learning the protocol.

A paramedic has a lot of responsibility. When you arrive at the scene of an emergency, you must know what to do right away. Can you imagine being injured, and as you lay bleeding, the medic pulls out a book and tries to figure out what treatment he/she needs to administer? I could easily understand why my instructor wanted us to know the protocol.

There are occasions when people have reactions to certain drugs that you might administer to them. When this happens, you must know what to give them to counteract that drug. You don't have time to pull your book out and do research. Adverse reactions to medicines can be life threatening. As a Paramedic, you respond to these runs to help people, but you can hurt them just as fast.

Now I'm starting to have a lot of fun in class. There were some things I already knew how to do. I learned the skills in the ER. I could start IVs. I could intubate. I could use a defibrillator (an electrical device used to counteract fibrillation of the heart muscle and restore a normal heartbeat by applying a brief shock). I was already good but now I'm better. My ego and my self-esteem have escalated. I feel as if I'm ready to save the whole world. I'm doing so much better in the second module than I did in the first. There is no way she is going to put me out of this class, unless I do something mighty drastic, or my grades fall past the minimum.

Just as I thought things were going smooth, the bottom fell out. In class, we had to demonstrate how to defibrillate if a person is in V-Fib or Ventricular Fibrillation. V-Fib is a condition when the heart is not beating, but it's just quivering. It needs an electrical shock to stimulate it to beat again. The defibrillator has two paddles that you use to administer the shock. It can be manually set to give so many Jules of electricity. When it was my turn to demonstrate the procedure, I went through it just fine. I reached down to turn the defibrillator off and mistakenly hit the recharge button. My instructor, who was standing close to me, asked me in a very stern voice, "What are you doing?" I said, "I'm trying to turn the defibrillator off." Picture this. I've got both defibrillator paddles in my hand. I turn toward her to respond to her question. I was aware that you were not to point the paddles at anyone, but I got nervous when she questioned me. I forgot that the paddles were in my hand as I was talking to her. She screamed at the top of her voice, "Don't point those paddles at me!" She slapped my hands so hard that I almost dropped the paddles. In anger I shouted back at her, "If you just tell me what I did wrong, maybe I can straighten it out!" She told the class, "This is what I'm talking about. Some of you are dangerous and you are going to kill people if I allow you to become paramedics! So, rest assured, you will not get out of this class unless I can be sure that you will operate safely in the field."

I'm still standing there, angry as I could be, saying to myself, "This woman just hit me!" She said, "Johnson, put the paddles in the defibrillator and discharge them." I did just as she asked, and the machine went off. This woman had tried everything possible to get me out of that class. I just gave it to her on a silver platter. Since I'm on my way out, I might as well make it good. I decided to mop the room up with her.

She is presently walking back and forth ranting and raving about the incident like a proud rooster. She struts with satisfaction at achieving her goal of getting rid of me. All my frustrations are coming to a climax! She has pushed me and embarrassed me for the last time. Since she struck a blow, it is time for me to strike a mightier one for all that has transpired through my struggles in this program. My expression reflected what I was thinking. As I walked toward her, two of my buddies ran to the front and grabbed me. They knew. They whispered in my ear, "Johnson don't do it. We only have three more weeks of class, and you are passing. She had to do something to get you out of here because she is desperate. She can't flunk you. If she could have, she would have already." "Don't give it to her that cheap. Come on with us back to your seat and cool off." Since I had come so far, I decided to listen to them. After she finished ranting, she said, "Now that I got that off my chest, we can move on with class."

Now comes the moment of truth. It's time to take finals. To take the Practical Exam, you had to pass the final exam with better than a 77% average. I received 89% on the written exam. Now, I qualify to take the Practical Exam. There are 10 skill stations set up that you must go through and pass to their satisfaction. The first thing we had to do was record a perfect CPR strip. Next, we had to defibrillate and intubate. She had the hardest station. At her station you had to do EKG recognition within five seconds. She would hand you 10 EKG strips, one at a time. You had to tell what the patient looked like with that rhythm and tell how you would treat him with basic and advanced life support. Her station was so critical that even if you passed all the rest, if you didn't pass her station, you flunked. The other medics were lined up at all the other stations. No one was at her station. I wonder why?

I went through all the stations with a breeze. I saved hers for last. I knew I had to go to that station. My heart was pounding, and I was sweating. I knew she had my life in the palm of her hands. I must keep a cool head and stay focused. I had the ability to succeed, but with all the knowledge and skills I have acquired, will this be enough to get me past her? I took a deep breath and with a slow and nervous walk, I moved toward her station. The two things that you need the most to pass her station are good EKG recognition and excellent knowledge of the protocol. I had excelled in both. In my mind, I'm wondering does she have me or do I have her?

When I walked in, she explained the rules and what she expected. She handed me my first rhythm. She said, "What is this?" I said, "It's a Bradycardia. This is a slow heart rhythm. She says, "What does the patient look like with this rhythm?" I said the patient may not display any symptoms or they may start to sweat and become short of breath. She asked me how I would treat the patient with that rhythm? I said, "If the patient was asymptomatic (which is without symptoms), I wouldn't do anything. If the patient were symptomatic, I would give them oxygen, and start an IV. If the heart rate fell below 50, then I would give them Atropine to pick the rhythm up. Then I would monitor their EKG very closely to make sure the heart rhythm does not get out of control." Next, she gave me some of the harder rhythms. I imagine she thought the ones she gave me were too simple. She says, "What is this?" I took one look at it and immediately said, "This is an idioventricular rhythm with multi-focal PVCs. This is a dying heart rhythm with extra beats that don't look alike because they are coming from different areas of the heart." Next, she says, "How does the patient look with this rhythm?" The look on her face was saying I've got him now. My reply was, "The patient is unconscious. The skin is cool and pale or ashen gray. Unless the heart is stimulated right away, the patient will surely die." She said, "What's the treatment?" I said, "The first thing we should do is start CPR. Then the patient should be intubated. Next, the patient should be given a series of cardiac drugs to try to rejuvenate the heart to a more acceptable rhythm. Depending on the rhythm, you can contemplate defibrillation."

She tried to throw me a curve by asking me auxiliary questions. But I was ready for her. She asked about various IV drip medications, and allergic situations, when people can't take the prescribed drug. My knowledge of the protocol was really coming through for me now. I answered all her questions with little room for doubt. I was supposed to interpret 10 strips. After I went through five, she said, "You can leave." My reply was, "I thought we had to do 10 strips?" She reiterated with a very firm but discouraged voice. "You can leave!" Despite her best efforts to flunk me, it became evident that I knew my protocol and how to read EKGs. In fact, I gave her a three-minute dissertation on each rhythm. I can't describe how I felt as I walked out of that room. As much as I disliked her, in my heart I really thanked her. Had she not been so hard on me, I probably would not have learned what I learned the way I learned it. When you learn things the hard way, they are not easily forgotten. You know what you know, and nobody can take it from you.

I felt that I had overcame the highest hurdle of my career in the medical profession. Now I could walk back to the ER with my head held up high. I could look all those nurses in the eyes who were waiting for me to fail. I could proudly say, "I did it." When I saw the other three African Americans come out of her room, they ran to me and said, "How did you do?" In my proudest voice I said, "I passed." They literally picked me up and swung me around. One of the guys kissed me on the cheek. They said, "We were so worried about you. It was obvious that she didn't want you to pass." There were 40 men that went into that class, including 16 African Americans and 24 Caucasians. Only 16 passed, four African Americans and 12 Caucasians. The war isn't over yet. Now it's time to take the state examination to become certified.

We had to drive to Indianapolis, Indiana to take a six-hour examination. The test was taken in two sessions. The first part was Anatomy, Physiology and Pharmacology. The second session was all situations that you take with a magic wand. The questions would read as follows: "You have an 85-year-old woman eating at a restaurant and she suddenly collapsed. You arrive on the scene. What would you do first?"

The answers would read like this:

1. Check her food tray.
2. Check her purse.
3. Check the patient.
4. Ask bystanders what happened.

Now you take the magic wand and pick the answer that you feel is best. Once you scroll over the answer with the wand, it will read out what the results are.

For instance, if you chose number one it would say, "Her food looks good, why don't you have some." If you chose number two it would say, "She has medication in her purse for high blood pressure and diabetes." That's how the wand would go. You had to choose the best answer. What we didn't know was that there was more than one good answer. If the question had three good answers and you only chose one, you gained five points, but you had 10 taken from you. You needed 700 points to pass the state exam. I only scored 460. My other buddies also failed. You can take the test three times. The next time I took the test, I scored 500. My other buddies also failed again. Then we found out from one of the other medics that was in our class that you could go to Indianapolis and review your test. They had the same problems we had. They had failed the test too.

Fred, Harold, and me got together to go to review our tests. This is when we found out about the magic wand. We were only checking one answer when there were two or three good answers. The next time we went back to retest, we all passed!

Now I'm a certified, bonafide, and stamped on both sides, para-medic! I feel like superman. I was ready. I was willing. I was able. With my skills, I was prepared to save the whole world. I went back to the ER but not the same person. This time I had a patch on my shoulder that said I was now a "Certified Paramedic." I wore it proudly. Those who doubted me could only look at me now with respect. The doctors applauded my success. All the hard work and the sacrifices I made have now paid off. This is what I was after.

I soon learned that the power of man is fleeting. With all my skills in saving lives, I didn't have the power over life or death. The only one that can save everyone is God. I soon found this out the hard way.

One week after I got my certification, they brought a man into the ER who was in full arrest. I said to myself, "Now I can imple-ment all the skills I have been taught." I said to myself, "Do some-thing! You were trained to save lives!" This was the first full arrest I'd encountered since I became a paramedic. I immediately jumped on the man's chest and started doing CPR. When I looked in his face, a thousand pains went through my heart. This was my best friend's father. He was very special to me because he taught me how to fish.

I will never forget our first-time fishing. His son didn't like to fish so he took me. I was afraid of worms. He took a worm out of the bucket and showed me how to put it on the hook. Then he said, "OK, now you do it." I put on a pair of gloves just to get the worm out of the pail, but I just couldn't put him on the hook. I said, "I know what I will do. I'll ask him to show me again how to put the worm on. This time I'll give him my pole. When he does, I won't have to bait my own hook."

I said Mr. Arnold, "Can you show me how to put this worm on my hook. I forgot what you showed me." He said, "No problem." He took my pole and put the worm on the hook. Then he said, "Did you see how I did it?" My reply was, "Yes." Then he took the worm off the hook and handed the pole back to me and said, "Now you put it on." The warm thoughts of him made me more anxious to save him because of our special bond. He taught me how to fish. Each time he went, he took me. The other medics took over doing CPR. I immediately looked at his EKG strip to interpret it. He was in asystole. This is just a straight line with no heart rhythm. The doctor grabbed the defibrillator and started to shock him. They shocked him several times, but the rhythm didn't change. I'm saying to myself, "This is your best friend's father! The man taught you how to fish! You have to save him!" I started checking his IV fluids, pushing meds through his IV, and anything else I could think to do.

His heart just wasn't responding. After 45 minutes of intensive resuscitation, the doctor finally said we couldn't save him, and to stop CPR. I said, "No Doc, don't stop! We have to keep going! This is my best friend's father!" I was yelling frantically. He said, "Dave, all efforts have failed. There is nothing else we can do." I immediately jumped on his chest and started doing CPR. I said, "Come on Doc, don't stop now. We have saved people before in full arrest situations. There must be something else you can do! I'll do CPR. Shock him! Give him some more medicine! Do something! Just don't stop!" He took a long look at me and in a very sad voice, with tears forming in his eyes, he said, "Dave, I'm sorry. I know he was your friend, but he's gone." Then he walked away.

I really started to berate myself. I was feeling what was the point of going to school to get all this training to save lives and when it's really put to the test, I can't save the ones I really want to save. His wife walked over to me. Tears were rolling down my face. How could I face her and tell her we couldn't save him when she was depending on me to help her. Instead of me consoling her, she was trying to console me. She said, "I just want to thank you. It was obvious you did all you could. I'm glad you were here."

As a child, I spent many nights at his house. I could reflect, when his son and I were kids and he caught us jumping up and down in the bed. He made both of us clean up the room. Once we were finished, he came in and tore it a part. Then, he said, "Now clean it up again." We put everything back together, feeling we were through. He came in and said, "Are you finished?" We said, "Yes. Is it ok this time?" He didn't say a word. He proceeded to tear it apart again. Then he said, "Clean it up again." He wasn't the kind of man you would want to argue with. He stood about 6'0" tall and weighed about 250 pounds. Yes, he was a big man with a big beer belly. After we cleaned things up again, we just sat quietly in the corner, afraid to say anything. He walked in and looked the room over. Our hearts just fell to the floor. He could see the tears in our eyes, as we looked at him, afraid that he was going to make us clean the room again. He started laughing and he laughed and laughed and laughed.

Then he said, "You kids look like convicts on death row who just had their names called. The reason I made you clean up this room over and over was to emphasize an important point. I wanted you to understand that it is hard to furnish a house. I can't afford to buy more beds. When you have decent beds, you need to take care of them." Then he said, "Now, will I have to get on you about jumping up and down on the bed again?" He received a unanimous, "Nooo!" Then he took us out for ice cream. On the surface, he appeared rough but deep inside was a nice man.

I sat quietly reflecting on this tragic event, thinking to myself, "If you can't save the ones you love, then whom can you save?" I walked out of the ER with my head down and tears running from my eyes. My head nurse came over to me and said, "Why don't you just take the rest of the day off?" This was a very humbling experience for me. I learned then that, just because I have acquired these lifesaving skills, I still didn't have the power to control who lived and who dies, not even the ones I love. As a paramedic, you will find that there will be times, even at your best, your best is not good enough. The children, the mothers, the fathers, the sisters, the brothers, they all belong to somebody. When their lives are in jeopardy, everyone is looking at the paramedic to save them. Nothing can bring you more joy than to give these loved ones back to their families. But nothing is more painful than to tell someone you couldn't save the life of his or her loved one. You learn that you are not God. You don't have the power of God. But, with the help of God, you can make a difference.

CHAPTER 7

NOW THAT I HAVE MADE IT - WHAT'S NEXT?

WELL, JUST WHEN I THOUGHT IT WAS SAFE TO GO back in the water, I soon found out I was facing a new set of problems. The Paramedic Program was new to the ER. Paramedics were trained in many procedures that the nurses weren't allowed to do. One procedure was intubations. The paramedics were allowed to give narcotics in the field. Even if they lost radio contact, if they stuck to the protocol, they could function independently. A nurse could never give a narcotic without a doctor's written or verbal order.

The nurses, on the other hand, could give paramedics permission to give a narcotic. Some of the nurses in the ER were becoming jealous of the paramedics. The problem started to escalate. The nurses were feeling threatened. When the paramedics would call in for permission to give a narcotic over the bio-phone (this was a two-way radio system that the paramedics used to stay in contact with the hospital while treating emergencies in the field), the nurses who answered the phone were refusing to give the medics permission. They were using excuses, such as they were not comfortable with the medic who was handling the call.

They were starting to question a lot of the things the paramedics were doing, especially in the ER. The nurse's felt that soon they would be phased out. The doctors had to call all the nurses in for a meeting. They shared with the nurses that they weren't replaceable. A paramedic can't do the job of a nurse. However, the nurses with the proper training can do a paramedic's job. Things soon quieted down and we were back to business as usual.

At first, I was just an active onlooker. Now I'm an active participant. My role in the ER had become more extensive. I became very good at starting IVs. I developed a technique that was so good I would only stick the patient one time. They would say, "Johnson, see if you can start an IV on that patient, we have tried but couldn't get in." Before I attempt to stick the patient, I carefully look around their hands and arms to find the best vein. After I have spotted the best vein, then it becomes a matter of technique.

To start an IV, you need sturdy hands, and good needle placement. Once you go in the vein with the needle, you bevel up so that you don't go through the vein. After you see the blood coming through, then you pull your needle out and then thread your catheter.

One evening, I was put to the ultimate challenge. Two Caucasian males came in by ambulance. They were working on a power line and got electrocuted. After the Doc examined them, he said to me, "See if you can start an IV on those two white guys in cubicle two. I'm going to call the burn unit in Chicago and talk to their team." When I went into the cubicle, I saw two Black men. I went back to Doc and said, "Where are the two white men? He said, "In cubicle two." I said doctor, "It's two black men in cubicle two." He said, "No, those are two white men. This is how they look when they have been hit with high voltage."

I went back in and did a thorough examination. The only thing white on them was the bottom of their feet. They were burned to a crisp. I had always heard this expression but seeing it for the first time really put the emphasis on it. Their skin looked like burnt meat. It was charcoal black, hard, and scaly. I looked good but there were no veins to be found anywhere. The two men were semi-conscious, they had airways in their mouths, and they were moaning in pain. Dr. Sims was on duty. He was a very good ER doctor. He had to do a cut-down (this is an emergency procedure that doctors use to start an IV). They make an incision on the lower limb to expose a vein, and then they thread an IV needle through it. After he got the IVs started, we managed to keep both patients alive until the ambulance came to transfer them to the Chicago Burn Center. We were told later that those two guys did not make it. Their burns were too extensive. I really felt sorry for those men. I knew that if they had survived, their quality of life wouldn't have been the same.

The doctors were not the only ones who were starting to have confidence in me. All my personal friends must have gotten the word that I was a paramedic now. My phone rang constantly.

These were some of the requests: "Hey Dave can you come over and look at my baby? I can't get her fever down." Or "Can you come over and look at my father or my mother? They don't look good." "Can you come by and check my blood pressure? I think it's up." "My little boy just fell and cut his head. Can you come and look at it to see if he needs stitches?" I soon found myself running day and night. My friends felt they had their own personal medic they could call for emergencies. But I loved it! When the call came in, I would put on my Superman cape and take off! Johnson to the rescue! Off I went! Duty calls!

Whenever I traveled out of state, I thought I would get a rest from being a medic. It seemed as if my friends were just waiting for me to get there.

I was immediately requested to go and check different ones. If an emergency came up, I was summoned to the area right away. Let me tell you what happened when I went to the home of a famous recording artist in Encino, California. My daughters were playing with their boys out by the pool and one of the boys fell and cut his hand. My daughters ran into the house and said, "Daddy, Marty cut his hand!" We looked toward the door as the other children walked in with Marty. His hand was bleeding. Everyone panicked. I immediately jumped up! I said, "Someone give me a towel!" I wrapped the towel around his hand to control the bleeding. After the bleeding was under control, I examined the cut. To my surprise, it was a small superficial cut on the thumb.

His grandmother said, "Do we need to take him to the emergency room?" My reply was, "No, all he needs is a few steri-strips. If you have some, I can fix him up as good as new. I've seen hundreds of wounds like these in the ER that we didn't have to suture." The grandmother said, "I don't have that item." I said, "Can we get it at the drugstore?" "Yes," she said. One of the brothers of the famous singing group had just bought a Rolls Royce. He gave his sister the keys and told her to take me to the store. Picture it. There were people camped outside their house. They were hanging on the fence and sleeping on the grass. They were just waiting to get a glimpse of the singers. We went to the drug store. I brought steri-strips, gauze, bandages, and ointment. After I fixed his hand, I became the hero of the week.

It seemed that wherever I traveled, I would end up using my skills to help someone. After working very hard that first year, I bought me a boat. I was invited to Minnesota to go fishing with my friend. While traveling on the interstate, my wife noticed a motorcycle lying on the ground and two people lying next to it. They were on the opposite side of the interstate. The first thing she said was, "Look, there is someone hurt! You have to stop and help them. I pulled my van over and ran to the other side of the interstate to see if I could help. As I approached the injured, I said, "I'm a paramedic, can I help!" The two attendees said, "Yes, please help!" There were two people lying on the ground, a man, and a woman. Their fellow riders were attending to them. They said, "The front tire blew out on their motorcycle, and they were thrown from the bike." The first thing we were taught to do as paramedics was to do an assessment (a one-minute survey to ascertain all injuries) and treat the worst ones first.

I went to the man. I explained to him that I was a paramedic. I was going to examine him briefly just to see what his injuries were. I didn't remove his helmet. I started with his head and worked my way down. He didn't complain of any pain until I touched the right side of his ribs. He also complained when I examined his abdomen and his right thigh in the femoral area. Right away, I knew the man might have fractured ribs that could have easily punctured the lung, a possible ruptured spleen in the abdomen and a possible fractured femur. Any one of these injuries could cause a patient to go into shock due to blood loss. Now that I know what is wrong with him, I told him to just lie still, and I was going to go check the woman.

I went to the woman and told her the same thing I told him. "I'm a paramedic and I want to examine you." The state trooper told me the ambulance was on the way. Her examination showed that she only had some bruises but nothing major. I told her to lie still. I was going back to her friend. The ambulance was on its way.

As I walked toward him, the ambulance pulled up. A young lady and a young man stepped out of the ambulance. I said,

"Which one of you is a paramedic?" Their reply was, "Neither, we are both EMTs." I knew right then that this would complicate matters because the gentleman was going to need some advance life support. He was a class three trauma. I said, "I'm Dave Johnson. I'm a paramedic from Indiana. I have assessed these people and this gentleman is a class three trauma, which makes this a load-and-go situation. Meaning he needs to be transported immediately to the closest facility." I said, "The man has a possible fractured rib, ruptured spleen, and fractured femur. The other patient has only minor scrapes and bruises." The young lady said, "We will have to examine them first." I said, "I don't mean any disrespect, but you are just EMTs. I'm a paramedic. What more will you find than what I just shared with you? While you are sitting here playing everything by the book this man may die." She responded, "Like I said, we have to examine them first."

She walked over to the man and tried to take his helmet off. Once they got his helmet off, they tried to take his jacket off by pulling on the sleeves. The patient screamed in pain. I interrupted and said, "Hold it! If you insist on undressing this man, let me show you how to take the jacket off." I said, "Sir, raise your hands above your head as much as you can." I told her, "Now grab the bottom of his jacket and roll it up under his back toward his head." I told the male EMT to hold traction on his neck. Once the jacket cleared his back, I told her to grab the sleeves and pull straight up. The jacket came right off. She did her 60-second survey and found the same injuries I had told her. I said, "Now will you get the man out of here." She said, "First I have to take his vitals."

Once again, I said, "Listen, this man has multiple traumas. If you don't get him out of here now his condition is going to turn critical!" She ignored me. She took his blood pressure. I said, "What did you get?" She says, "110/70." I knew that wasn't his blood pressure. The man's color was pale. His breathing was shallow. He was panting to breathe. His skin was cool and moist. These were all the classic signs of shock. Hemorrhagic shock (shock due to blood loss). I said, "Let me take his blood pressure." She refused but I insisted. The man's blood pressure was 80/60. His level of consciousness was starting to diminish. I became frantic at this point. I told the guy, "Give the man oxygen!" He proceeded to give the man oxygen.

She was taking the bed and spine board out of the ambulance. As he held traction on the man's head, she put a C-collar on the patient's neck. They were trying to log roll him on the spine board. The patient screamed again. I assisted them getting him on the board. I helped them put him on the bed. She then started to tie the man's head down to the spine board with Kerlex. I said, "Listen, by the time you get to the hospital you are going to have a good-looking corpse! The things you are doing are fine but not in a critical situation like this! You are worried about the man's spine but it's not going to help him if he bleeds to death!"

I asked the guy, as we were putting the man in the ambulance, "Who is in charge?" He said, "She is." I asked if he could patch me into the hospital where they were taking him ? He did. I told the nurses, "I have a patient who is a class three trauma and I need to speak to the ER doctor right away." The doctor answered the Bio-phone. He said, "This is the ER doctor, go ahead." I said, "This is Paramedic Dave Johnson from Indiana. While traveling on the interstate I witnessed an accident with two motorcyclists. Their front tire blew out at about 50 miles per hour. He and his rider were thrown from the bike. He is a class three trauma who is going into shock. He has a possible hemo-pneumothorax (a punctured lung) and possibly a ruptured spleen; his abdomen is rigid and tender to the touch and a possible fractured femur. I've been on the scene since the onset, and I can't get the EMTs to treat this man as a class three trauma. She has been doing everything by the book but in the process the man is dying." He said, "Put her on!" I could hear him tell her to get that man in there stat!

She was angry! Her face was cherry red. She screamed at her partner reaffirming to him that she was in charge. She told him, "Get the lady and let's go!" The lady rider was already standing and watching what was going on. He immediately grabbed the lady, walked her to the rig, strapped her in and they took off. They didn't leave before the young lady walked up to me and called me a "Butt hole" before getting into the ambulance. I told her that she was in the wrong field. "If you want to dress things up you need to get into the clothing business." His friends told me they were on their way to the Indy 500 when the accident happened. They thanked me over and over for stopping to help. The state trooper told me that she was also glad I stopped because they were taking too much time and that this man could have very easily died. She took my name and address. We all shook hands, and I went back to my vehicle. My wife said, "How did it go?" I said, "Sit back, this is going to be a long story."

As we were driving, I was thinking to myself, "I really hope those medics get to the hospital safely and that they are able to save this man." Those medics sent to the scene of that accident need to be retrained. It's obvious they don't have a clue as to what to do when they encounter trauma. I told my wife on the return trip, "If we have an accident and those two medics show up, don't let them touch me, just call me a cab."

I'm really beginning to understand the seriousness of this job. Being a paramedic is more than just walking around in your uniform bragging that you are a paramedic. The question is, can you do the job?

As a paramedic I had to attend many seminars for extra training. These were valuable learning experiences. I met other paramedics from other parts of the state of Indiana. It was obvious they were proud of their profession. Many of them had so many patches on their uniforms they looked like Raggedy Ann dolls. There were paramedics that had belts laced with every piece of equipment you can carry on a belt. They had their cars decaled with all kinds of blue lights, license plates, stickers, and every other paramedic paraphernalia. When they got out of their cars, they looked like RoboCops. They had so much gear on, they could barely move around.

I agree that a paramedic should look the part, but I found that looks could be deceiving. Some paramedics looked so polished, prepared, and exuded so much confidence. They looked like they could save the world but some are as worthless as tits on a bull. I may be a bit graphic by saying this, but I will explain why. When you see these paramedics get out of their rigs with pins, awards and trophies and patches all over their chests, don't be disillusioned to believe that this is a very skilled paramedic. Being a paramedic is not about how many patches you wear on your chest or how much equipment you can carry on your belt. It's about can you do what you must do when it's time to do it.

For years I have loved track and field. I would go to the state track meet every year. I will never forget a young kid I saw who was about to run the 100-meter dash. The other kids had on nice colorful warm-ups and track shoes. This kid had on an old dingy uniform. His shoes were so dirty, you couldn't see the white on them. As I looked at his feet, I noticed that he didn't have on any socks. His hair was braided but it wasn't neat. The other kids were taking short sprints, trying to get ready for the race. He just stood there with his hands on his hips. He didn't do any warming up. He appeared very unconcerned about the others. I said to myself,

Look at that little raggedy kid. I bet those guys are going to burn him up on that track. Boy was I ever wrong! When the gun went off, that kid set the track ablaze! I said, "Will you look at that?" We all judged this kid by his appearance as to what his talents were going to be. This is what I meant about the difference between appearance and performance.

There was a doctor that we worked with in the ER that was fresh out of Medical School, and he looked good. He had a nice, neat hair cut with a part on the side. He was neatly shaven and had on good-smelling cologne. His medical jacket was pure white and nicely pressed. His slacks were pressed, and his shoes were shined. Yes, he was the epitome of what a doctor should look like. I might add, there is nothing wrong with that. Whatever you profess to be, you should look the part. When I was out there, my uniform was always neat. But don't be deceived by thinking that a person's appearance reflects his skills or abilities. This doctor didn't know how to suture. In fact, he couldn't treat half the emergencies that came through the door. We had to lead him around like a child.

In comparison, we called in a surgeon for a gunshot wound to the chest. When this thoracic surgeon came through the doors of the ER, he looked like he hadn't shaved in a week. His suit was wrinkled. His shoes were dull and scuffed. He had a scowl on his face as if someone had just taken his money. Your first impression of this doctor might be that you wouldn't want him working on you. But, to watch him work was something to behold! This guy had skills. He was smooth. He knew his way around the body like a mechanic around a car. The patient crashed on us. This doctor did a cut-down. Put in a chest tube. Put a sub-clavian tube in the patient's neck. He cracked the man's chest and manually massaged his heart. It became obvious that there was nothing related to trauma that this doctor couldn't do. So, when you compare the two, Wally Cleaver of Leave It to Beaver and Oscar Madison from the Odd Couple, who would you have chosen?

I worked with a paramedic that was very good in tough situations. His nickname was Happy. They called him that because he was always smiling. He didn't have anything on his belt. In fact, he didn't even wear a belt. He was scruffy looking. Despite his appearance, he was one of the best. Picture this. There is a bad accident on the highway, and it's pitch dark outside. There is a car turned over in a ditch. There are people laying everywhere, and you have trauma up to your ears. You must crawl down into the ditch, holding your pen light in your mouth for light, to start an IV before someone expires. Happy is the man you want on the scene. He was so cool in trauma situations. Nothing ruffled his feathers. The worse things got, the better he worked. When he had to go down into the trenches, he came out with IVs started and bleeding controlled.

Don't equate a person's looks with his level of performance. If you do, you might end up very disappointed. Don't be so quick to assume because he looks good that he is good. There are many great paramedics across the country; if you get injured, I hope you manage to get one of them.

The emergency room I worked in was a training center for the new interns getting out of medical school. They had to work throughout the hospital, but they loved coming to the ER. Most of them had no trauma skills. Some couldn't start IVs. I showed many of them the proper way to suture. This came from my training when I first started in the ER. I was taught by some of the best. Many of the interns would say, "Boy you are so good. Why don't you go to medical school?" I told them I had my opportunity but at the time I couldn't cash in on it. Maybe if I didn't have a family, I would consider it.

There was one medical student who came to the ER for the summer that everyone loved. We hit it off right from the start. He was tall, slim, and good-looking. He had a warm, friendly personality. He was young and aggressive. It was obvious that he was going to make a fine doctor. Everywhere he went, I went right with him. I tried to show him everything I'd learned about emergency medicine.

Gerald also taught me a lot of things he had learned in medschool. We had a good time together, so much so that we started to go out socially. As our friendship flourished, the nurses noticed that we were always together. We became "boyz." We went to all the hospital parties. We even double-dated.

One day, he called me at home. He said, "Hey J, how about going on a blind date?" My reply was, "No, I hate blind dates. I'm always stuck with someone I don't want to be with." He said, "Ah come on J, just this one time." I said, "How does she look?" He very cautiously said, "I don't know, I've never seen her before. But she is my girlfriend's sister, who is home for spring break. She has been away at school that is why I haven't seen her." I said to myself, "Doc has always had good taste in women because he has always liked the ones that I liked." Currently in my life, I was going through a divorce. I said, "OK Doc. I'm going to try this just this once. I hope I don't get disappointed." He said, "I'll tell you what if she is pretty, we'll split the bill 50-50. If she is not, I'll pay for the whole thing."

He came by to pick me up in his new black BMW. We went to the south suburbs of Illinois to this very nice home. After we rang the doorbell, a very attractive woman answered the door. I said, "You must be my date!" She said, "I'm the mother. But the girls are ready, come on in." I started giving Doc a high five. If the mother looks that good, I know I'm in for a real treat.

We sat in the living room. I'm so excited. There is a big smile on my face, anticipating my date. Shortly, a lovely young lady walked around the corner. I said, "You must be my date!" Gerald spoke up right away and said, "Oh, no that's mine!" By now I'm frantic! I can barely wait to see this gorgeous woman come around the corner. I envisioned this beautiful model-type entering the room, but the reality was a 200-pound, medium-height woman with thick-rimmed glasses. As she opened her mouth to greet me, I was stunned by this rough course voice that said, "I'm your date." I tried all I could to hide my disappointment. I looked at Doc and he started laughing and couldn't stop. We introduced ourselves. She said, "I'm Gail, how are you?" I thought, "You don't want to know." I said, "Fine, I'm Dave." On the way to the door, Gerald leaned to my ear and said, "I've got dinner."

We went to a fine restaurant. I was surprised. We had great conversation. She lived in Atlanta, Georgia, and she was in her last year of medical school. We were having such a good time that we left Doc and his friend and went upstairs to the bar. Gerald came upstairs and called me to the door. He said, "J, you don't have to pretend that hard, I'm going to pay for dinner." I said, "You know Doc, I don't mind going half because I'm really having a nice time." We struck a chord because we both liked medicine. I learned that they were half-sisters and she lived with her father. This is one occasion that I learned a lesson from my own words. "Don't judge people by their appearance." She was a very nice person, and intelligent with very stimulating conversation.

When we took the ladies home, I gave her a nice hug and kiss. I even got her number so that when I was in her hometown, I could look her up. She told me she would show me the town.

One afternoon, Gerald and I were working together in the ER. We were standing in the hall discussing a patient when in through

85

the door came a beautiful, young lady with dark hair and hazel eyes. We both stopped talking at the same time. Our eyes fell upon this young lady, and as she walked past, we both said, "Wow! Who is that?" She wore a pair of Sassoon Jeans. Boy did she look good in those jeans! This girl had an hour-glass figure.

She was a vision of loveliness as she walked past. We eyed her from head to toe. We noticed the sound of her clicking heals as she gracefully walked in a pair of white cowboy boots. The boots accented a western top with the fringes hanging off the sleeves. This was a perfect combination that was tucked neatly in the waist of the jeans. She wore a wide belt, with a large buckle, that lay neatly at her waist. As she walked, you could see the name, Sassoon, sway as her body shifted from side to side in the designer jeans. She walked up to one of the nurses and asked for one of the technicians. Someone told her that the technician was in the ER. They informed her that the technician had just left. She turned and walked back past us, giving us another visual of what we had just beheld. Again, our eyes followed her all the way out the door. Right away Doc said, "I'm going to find out who that is." I said, "If I find out first you won't."

I worked a double shift because someone had called in. The technician and this young lady came back to the ER that evening. The technician, Betty, and this beautiful young lady were good friends. Betty was introducing her to some of the people on the evening shift. The girl was a new employee to the hospital. She lived across from the hospital, in the dorm. At that time, the hospital housed the residents and exchange students. She was going to school to be an Electro Diagnostic Technician. These are people that do the brain wave test, checking for seizures, brain tumors, etc. Betty was an Electro Diagnostic Technician too. That is how they became friends. I knew that when I saw Gerald, he was going to be disappointed. You see, Betty was infatuated with Gerald, and he knew it. There was no way that Betty was going to let him talk to her friend. So, that left Doc out of the picture. When I told him, he looked so sad. But the door was wide open for me.

I told Betty that I wanted to meet her friend. She related the message. Sherri gave Betty her number for me to call her in the dorm. I called her one evening. We had a great conversation.

There was a concert coming that weekend in Chicago. The music group, Earth, Wind and Fire was performing. I invited her to go. She accepted. We had a great time at the concert. We left and went to the after party at the "Cinderella Rockefeller Nightclub." This is when I learned that Sherri could really dance. I thought I had hit the jackpot with this young lady. Little did I know I was sitting on a piece of dynamite! I gave her my numbers to call me at work in the mill. At that time, I had an office job. She didn't just call once or twice or three times. She called every five minutes. I would say, "Look, I'm going to the bathroom, I'll call you back." She said, "That's ok I'll hold on." This went on all week. She would also be sitting at the gate when I got off work. As I exited the Mill, the joy of the vision that I first beheld was diminishing into a dread. She wanted me to spend time with her every day. I had no time to myself. We only dated. This was not a full-blown relationship. What did I get myself into?

When I worked in the ER, she spent a lot of time there. If she wasn't talking to me, she was talking to my best friend Gerald. I told Gerald that I was going out of town on the weekend but don't tell Sherri. When I returned, Betty approached me and asked me if Gerald and I went out of town together? My response was, "Gerald was still here. I went out of town." She says, "Have you talked to Sherri?" I said, "No, what's going on?" She says, "Sherri said she was going to Gerald's apartment, but she never came back to the dorm. I called her the entire weekend, but she was not there." I called Gerald. I asked him, "How was your weekend?" He said, "Oh, it was fine." I said, "Did you have any company?" His response was, "Sherri came by. She was upset that you were out of town, and she didn't have anyone to talk to." I asked him, "How long did she stay?" He said, "Well, I gave her some wine and she drank too much so I suggested that she sleep on the sofa and not try to drive home that night." Gerald might have suspected that I wasn't buying all of that. It was too well written.

I told Gerald, "Let me clear the air for you. Whatever happened, I'm not upset. So, you can be honest with me. This will not affect our friendship." He said, "Are you sure J?" I said, "Yes, you can tell me the truth." He said, "Well she did drink too much. Since I knew I wouldn't have a chance with her, I just took advantage of the situation since she was upset with you." I said, "Ok my dear friend, she is your lady now." He said, "Are you sure J?" I said, "I'm sure. I just didn't know how to break it off without hurting her feelings. She has been driving me nuts."

Then I called her. I asked her the same questions I had asked Gerald. Her response was, "Gerald's mother was there. She encouraged me to stay the night since I had too much to drink." I said, "Did you sleep with my friend?" She hesitated. Then she says, "David please don't be mad. I had too much to drink and I wasn't myself." My response was, "I'm not angry. Since you like Gerald that much, you can continue to see him." She will never know how relieved I was. Betty was furious! She quit speaking to Sherri and Gerald. A week later, Gerald called me in the mill and said, "J, I should have listened to you. This girl is about to drive me nuts. She calls me all day long. She keeps my pager screaming. When I'm on the phone with her, she don't want to hang up." I laughed and laughed and said, "Gerald, didn't you think there was something wrong when I gave her up so easily?" He said, "Yes, I did? But now what should I do?" I said, "I'm sure you will figure something out." In my heart, I felt this was his punishment for not being a loyal friend. Despite this incident, we continued to be good friends.

When people work together for a long while they get to know each other very well. It was no different in the ER. We worked hard saving lives. At the end of the shift, many times we would end up at a party at one of the worker's homes. It seemed that everyone enjoyed a good party. Even though we all came from different backgrounds and different sections of town, we still had a commonality that started in the ER. There were no racial differences. The Blacks would go the White sections of town and the Whites would come to the Black sections of town. Those in the middle, the Indians the Mexicans, the Filipinos, and the Puerto Ricans would go wherever there was a party. I can't over-emphasize the fact that we partied! After all the blood and guts, all somebody had to say was, "There's a party over here!" We would all show up.

The one thing they all had in common was that everybody loved to drink. No one loved to drink more than Happy. Once Happy became full of alcohol and he just wanted to go to sleep. Not just on the sofa or in a chair, but in a bed. He would leave the party area and search through the house to find the bedrooms. Then he would take off all his clothes, down to his underwear, and climb into bed. We wouldn't miss him until the party was over. Someone would say, "Where is Happy?" We would all say, "Let's check the bedrooms." And 100% of the time that is where you would find him. One night, we went to the suburbs to one of the nurse's homes for a party after work. She said my husband is at work so my home is open. We went out there and boy did we have a good time. She had a brand-new home that I think she just wanted to show off. About 11 p.m. she said, "Party is over. I got to

get you guys out of here before my husband comes in at midnight."
We had such a good time. We left and went our separate ways.
When I arrived home, my phone was jumping off the hook. When
I answered, the woman was hysterical. I recognized the voice. It
was the nurse whose home we just left. I said, "Jessica, what's the
problem? She said, "David, please come back! Happy is in my bed
and I can't get him out! We were having so much fun we forgot to
check for 'Happy.'

I jumped into my car. I drove like a maniac back to her house.
I was hoping that I could get there before her husband. I rushed in.
She took me upstairs. There was Happy lying on his side in a fetal
position, sleeping like a newborn baby. I grabbed Happy by one
arm, and she grabbed the other. I reached to the floor and picked
up his clothes. We both practically drug him down to my car. We
threw him into the back seat, and I threw his clothes on top of him.
I took off! Just as I turned the corner from her house, her husband
was turning the corner in his truck, heading home. I drew a sigh of
relief. We had just missed him. I had met the man before at other
parties. He wasn't friendly, to say the least. Can you imagine what
would have happened if he had found Happy upstairs in his bed
without any clothes?

Happy was harmless. He wouldn't hurt a fly. He never tried to
talk to any of the ladies. He just liked to party and drink. When
he had too much, he wanted to go to bed wherever he was. That
can be just as dangerous as trying to drive home drunk. There were
so many other parties after that one. But before we left, we made
sure we had 'Happy' with us.

CHAPTER 8

A NIGHT TO REMEMBER

EVEN THOUGH I HAD GAINED A GREAT DEAL OF knowledge as a paramedic, I still didn't have any street smarts. Knowing absolutely nothing about running the streets or the people in them, I took everything at face value. I was raised in a very strict home. I was married a year after high school. My father explained life to us. He never let us associate with the "fast girl" that lived on our street. We had to be in the house when night fell. I had five brothers and one sister. My parents were hard-working people who wanted us to succeed in life. They felt that letting us get involved in the street life would ruin all of that. The mistakes I'm going to tell you about were strictly due to inexperience.

One of the ladies I worked with at the hospital had a sister that worked at the mill. She introduced us one day when her sister was at the hospital visiting. We had a friendly conversation. Olivia was about 5'6" or 5'7" tall. She was thick. She wasn't fat but she had big hips and big legs. She had a warm, friendly smile that was so inviting. We enjoyed each other's company right away. I learned that we didn't work far from each other in the mill. The job I had at that time allowed me to move freely around the plant. I went to Olivia's department to see her several times. We later became good friends. We had lunch together quite often.

She invited me to her apartment for a home-cooked meal. She bragged about being one of the world's greatest cooks. Since I knew she was married, I declined her invitations. She told me her husband worked a distance away at another mill. Once he arrived at work he'd never turn around and come back home. I just did not feel comfortable going to her apartment. Her sister that worked with us also lived in the same apartment building. She said if I came over for breakfast, she would call him at work to confirm his whereabouts. I wanted to sample her cooking, even though I was nervous about being in her apartment. Finally, she convinced me.

We both had the day off. I went to her apartment. She made the phone call as she said she would. Everything appeared to be just fine. She cooked a fabulous breakfast. We had sausage, bacon, eggs, toast, ham, hash browns, fruit, juice, and coffee. She topped it off with homemade biscuits. It was a smorgasbord! There was no doubt in my mind that she could cook.

After breakfast we sat on the sofa, engaged in conversation, when suddenly I heard a key in the door. My heart fell to my feet. The door slowly opened. I looked at her face. The big smile had given way to terror. Her mouth fell wide open as this big man walked into the room. My first instinct was to run, but he was standing in front of the door. When she spoke, I knew right away it was her husband. She said, "Honey what are you doing home? Did you forget something?" He never took his eyes off me as he spoke. He said, "Who is this man?" Her reply was, "This is Glenda's friend." This was her sister that lived upstairs. I held my hand out to shake his hand. Nervously I said, "Hello, how are you?" Then I said to Olivia as I set the stage for my exit, "Tell your sister this is the second time that I came over here to see her and she wasn't home." He never reached to shake my hand, so I tried to walk around him. I was so scared that he was going to hit me. For some unknown reason he let me leave. But he watched me all the way out the door. I was saying to myself, "If I could just get to my car, I will never do this again." Some lessons are short-lived. A couple of months later, they bought a house. They had a housewarming party after they were settled in their new home. She informed me that he was a jealous man, and the phone call made him suspicious. She assured him that I was Glenda's friend. Then she asked me if I would like to come to the housewarming party. My response was, "Don't you think he may get upset if he sees me there?" She said, "He probably doesn't remember what you look like. Just come in and blend in with the crowd. He won't notice you." Even though I was apprehensive, I still went to the party. Then, 10 minutes after I had arrived, Olivia came to me and said, "David I'm sorry. My husband told me to tell you to leave." Not fully understanding why I had to leave, I said, "I just got here. What did I do wrong." Her reply was, "You did nothing wrong. He said if I didn't ask you to leave, he would. I really preferred that I do it."

This presents a problem for me. My wife and I had just reconciled for the moment. To get out to go to the party, I had to come up with a story that would keep me out all night. Then, 10 minutes into the night and I have no place to go? What will I do for the rest of the night? I can't go home. I should have stayed at home. Plan A had failed. I had to come up with a Plan B. I noticed one of the ladies that worked in registration at the party. Previously, on several occasions she had invited me to her apartment to socialize. Never accepting her invitations before, I thought quickly. I wasn't attracted to her at all. But I'm desperate now. All I wanted was a place to cool out until morning.

I wasn't looking for anything physical. I figured we would just talk and get to know each other a little better. I went to her and told her I had to leave. I asked her if she would like some company when she left the party. Annie seemed very excited that I asked and said, "Yes!" I got her apartment number. I asked her, "About how long will you be here?" She said, "Oh, a couple of hours." I left. Not having any place to go, I decided to ride around the city to kill time. It's funny how time moves so slowly when you are watching it. I went from one end of the city to the other. Looking at my watch, I had only been out for about 30 minutes. So, I rode some more. I was bored. Steadily telling myself that I should have stayed at home. I went back to Olivia's house and parked down the street so I could see the people coming out of the party. I sat for so long I fell asleep. When I woke, guess who was coming out of the house – Annie. I was so glad to see her leaving. She walked down the street to a car with one of her co-workers. They were conversing as they opened the doors and continued chatting until the closing of the door and the starting of the car engine silenced their voices.

Annie was a nice girl, but since I considered myself in the fast lane now, she was just a little too slow for me. I followed them to the apartment. The girl dropped Annie off and left. I parked my car and went back to the door I saw Annie go into. I went up the steps to the main entrance of the apartment building. I walked down the hall to the apartment number that was written on the paper. Knocking on the door, I was surprised by a man's voice as he spoke from the other side of the door and said loudly, "Who is it!" Fear just rippled through my body. No one ever mentioned anything about Annie being married or having a boyfriend. I thought maybe this is her brother. So, I said, "Is Annie home?" The voice said, "Just wait right there!" Not realizing what he meant, I stood there like an idiot waiting. This is what inexperience in the streets will get you. Something told me you had better leave. I started backing away from the door when I noticed it opening. The nose of a shiny pistol poked through the crack first. I took off running! This man

94

fired a shot at me! The bullet went through the glass window in the door of the main entrance. I jumped from snow-covered steps. I was so afraid; I was running in mid-air until I touched the streets. The man fired again! I was running so fast trying to get to my car that when I reached it, I slid on the ice right past it. My heart was pumping fast. Exhaustion and fear had completely overtaken me. I was unwittingly in a life-or-death situation. Jumping to my feet, I grabbed the door to my car, jumped in and sped off!

So much for Plan B. What puzzled me more than anything else was why she would invite me to her apartment when she knew someone was there. I could have easily been shot or killed. I still needed somewhere to go. I couldn't go home. I thought about Glenda. I knew she lived alone. We were the best of friends. I felt that she would help me. It was about 3 a.m. The front entrance to her apartment was locked. I proceeded to go to the back of the building and up the stairs to the third floor. It was cold and windy. The back of the building didn't have a porch. There were only the narrow stairs leading to the doors. Outside there were garbage cans sitting in a small corner area next to the back door. Each apartment had its own small light over the door. As I stood outside, the wind ripping through my leather coat, I rubbed my cold, stiff hands together and knocked on the door.

Glenda came to the door. She peeked out the curtain and, recognizing it was me, she opened the door. "David, what in the world are you doing here at 3 a.m. in the morning?" she said. My reply was, "Your sister's husband put me out of his house shortly after I arrived. I asked Annie did she want some company and she invited me over. A man answered her door and shot at me. I barely escaped with my life." She says, "That was Annie's husband. Why would she tell you to come over there?" I said, "Glenda I need a place to cool out for the rest of the night. Can I rest here on your couch? She says, "Sure come on in." While she was getting me a blanket and a pillow, I sat on the couch pulling off my shoes. I told her, "I sure appreciate you letting me stay. You are a good friend." Suddenly, I heard this voice come out of her bedroom that said, "Who did you just let in this house?" Glenda said, "That's just Olivia's friend Dave. He just wants to cool out here for the night." The man said in a very angry voice, "You should not let any man in this house while I'm here! I should get up and shoot both of you!" Immediately, I started putting my shoes on. Glenda was trying to calm him down, but to no avail. I eased out the door and was down the steps in no time.

Where do I go from here? I'm running out of options. I thought about Lutheran General Hospital. The men's locker room has a bench. I knew how to get into the hospital after hours. I quietly secured entry through the security entrance and went to the locker room. No one was there. I'm very tired now. My body is aching from the cold weather, all the running for my life and the fear that had made my bones weak. Lying down, I fell fast asleep.

Suddenly the door opened. In the doorway stood one of the security officers. It would have to be the officer that disliked me, because he thought I was after his girlfriend that worked in the ER. I knew his girlfriend liked me, but I never talked to her, because I knew he was seeing her. In a very stern voice he said, "Johnson what are you doing here?" My reply was, "Man you won't believe the kind of night I'm having. I just want to cool out here until daybreak and I'll leave." He said, "Not on my shift. Either you leave now, or you are going to jail." So, I got up and went to my car.

It was about 5 a.m. in the morning. I decided to go to a Chicago suburb pancake house for breakfast. All the excitement of the past night has really given me an appetite. I ordered a big breakfast. When the waitress came back with the food, I was slumped over, head down on the table, drooling at the mouth and probably snoring. She says, "Sir you must have had a bad night." I said, "Lady if you only knew." Finally, I went home. I made a vow to myself that I would never let myself get caught up in a situation like that again.

Many people think that medical professionals lead dull lives. I am here to tell you that my life was anything but dull. Social analysts have said that people who have stressful jobs will need an outlet to relieve the stress. That's why many professional people with stressful jobs engage heavily in alcohol, sex, or drugs. I realize now why many of my coworkers were so heavily involved in those things.

CHAPTER 9

NOW I HIT THE STREETS

AFTER WORKING IN THE ER FOR A GOOD WHILE, I decided I was ready to take my skills to another level. The medics who came in on the ambulance seemed to have a lot of fun. I had never worked on the streets, but I always had the desire. One day, I asked one of the guys if I could come and ride on the ambulance. He said, "No problem, all you have to do is come down to the station and sign a waiver releasing the city of any responsibility and you can ride."

I knew exactly whom I wanted to ride with. Dick was my man. Dick and I worked together in the ER. Remember we called him 'Slick Dick.' He was always so cool. He was a veteran in the war to save lives. Dick was a very good medic. All the doctors praised his work as a paramedic on the ambulance. We had many memories of experiences we shared in the ER. I'll never forget the big woman that was bitten in the breast by the little lady or when we went to the psych unit for the CODE SEVEN. I looked forward to riding with him. Dick took his work very seriously. He gave me a little pep talk before he took me out on the ambulance. He said, "Johnson, everyone I pick up is not just some face in the crowd. I look at them as if they were my mother, father, brother, sister, or kids. Whatever you do, always treat the people right. Even though they may not be related to you, they still belong to someone who cares if that person lives or dies. If we picked up someone in your family, you would want us to give them the very best of care. So always give them your best. Don't mistreat people because you have the power to do so. Some of the medics use this job as a tool to mistreat people."

When I was a paramedic working on an ambulance, I soon learned what Dick had meant. A car hit a child. He was about six years old. When I arrived on the scene, the child lay in the street bleeding from his head. He was crying and calling for his mother. The bystanders said the child was playing with the other children and ran in the street to get a ball. We put the child on the spine board, strapped his head down and put him in the ambulance. The boy's mother pulled up as we were working on him. It is the instinct for any parent to get nervous seeing an ambulance in front of their house. Your first instinct is to run to the ambulance and see who is in there. Once you discover it's your child, naturally you panic, which is what the lady did. She climbed into the ambulance screaming, trying to get close to her child. One of the medics didn't want the lady back there so he proceeded to push her out of the ambulance. She started screaming, "That's my baby! That's my baby!" Without any feeling he said, "I don't care, we are working, you will have to wait outside." This is the uncaring feeling that Dick was talking about. I immediately stopped what I was doing. I called the lady and told the medic to let her in. His reply was, "She'll be in our way!" I said, "If this was your baby where would you want to be? There is nothing stronger that the bond between a mother and her children." I told the mother that if she would sit there on the side and allow me to try and help her son, she could stay. She agreed she would not get in our way. When we got the baby to the hospital the mother hugged my neck and thanked me for allowing her to be with her baby. The babysitter let them outside to play.

The last thing she expected to see when she arrived home was an ambulance. I told my medic companion on our way back to the station that he was never to put anyone out of the rig without my approval. I'm in charge at each scene and unless I tell him to put someone out, they can come along with the patient. He did not like what I said but when I'm in charge no one will ever be mistreated.

In my 20 years as a paramedic, I have observed many people that used their job to demean, to persecute, and to cause pain or express personal prejudices or feelings. There are many medics out on the streets picking up people every day that are as socially biased as they can be. Some of them hate kids, senior citizens, poor people, and ethnic groups, to say the least. The only reason some of them want to become medics is to be able to run up and down the streets with sirens blasting, running through stop signs and stop lights. There is something about going through lights that seems to give these young people a charge. Some are so morbid, and they seem to enjoy seeing people broken up or injured. They like the idea of being able to wear a uniform with decals and patches all over them. They enjoy working with all the lifesaving equipment that is used to save lives. But, as far as having empathy for people, some of them miss the mark.

One such person was Clark. Clark was medium-height, and kind of stocky. He had medium-brown, straight hair, with a thick mustache. He always wanted to ride with me. He said he liked the way I worked in the field. We were sent on a 703. This is the Fire Departments Code for a man down. As we entered the home, we observed a young lady lying on the floor. I asked the mother what happened. She was so upset we got very little information out of her. The patient was breathing, with no obvious signs of injury. I told Clark to go and get the bed. We were going to take this patient to the hospital. The girl was about 250 pounds. She was heavy.

The first thing out of Clark's mouth was, "I'm not picking up this fat woman!" Her family became irate. I tried to calm them down. I told Clark, "We can always call for extra help." His reply was, "Then you guys can get her. I'm not picking up her big bleep, bleep!" It took all I had to keep her family off Clark. They were incensed by his lack of tact, in an emergency. I might also add that this was his chosen profession, helping people in emergency situations. Size, creed, or color is not a factor when someone is sick. The girl's brothers helped me put her on the bed and into the ambulance. I made Clark get in the ambulance so he could drive us to the hospital. Clark drove like a maniac! He ran through stoplights and stop signs. I had to make him stop the ambulance. I told him, "If you have a death wish that is just fine! But don't take us with you!"

After we got to the hospital, I pulled Clark into a room by himself. He said, "I know you are upset with me, but I'm not hurting my back picking up these big heavy people because they allow themselves to get as big as a house." I said, "Clark, everyone in the world is not 120 pounds. Our job is not to draw conclusions or tell people how to live. Our job is to treat the emergency. You cannot express how you feel while you are on the scene. If you continue with this kind of conduct, I can assure you, you will have a very short life." After that experience, I never allowed him to ride with me again. It wasn't long before he was fired for mistreating patients.

Fortunately, this does not represent the majority. But like anything else, it only takes one or two to ruin the reputation that others work so hard to maintain. I've noticed the same trend working in the ER with the nurses and doctors. Some are only in the profession for money. I've seen them let people lie on the beds and suffer, while they sit and smoke their cigarettes and talk about the latest soap opera. Some nurses have refused to give patients something as simple as a glass of water. There have been those who refused to pick up the phone and call the patient's doctor to get medicine to help alleviate their pain. I personally heard some of them say, "Let them hurt. It serves them right." There were nurses in the ER who would let elderly people stand near their loved ones for hours without offering them a chair. How could people be so cruel to the elderly?

I've seen medics toss elderly people around like sacks of potatoes. It's obvious that there are many in the medical profession that don't have sympathy or empathy for the sick. They are in the wrong profession. The medics I have trained were told right from the start that the greatest thing you can give a patient is to let them know that you care. There are many people in the medical profession that practically give their lives for the profession. It's not about money or making a name for yourself. So how do you weed out those that don't really have the love of the profession? By this I mean, when you see someone who is obviously on the job for the glory, or there to inflict his or her personal feelings on people, what do you do? What I did was to be the best that I could be. When I could make a difference, I tried. Those who were doing things that were unacceptable soon fired themselves.

I remember one evening, an elderly lady came in using a cane. The nurse put her on a bed and gave her a gown to put on. This nurse had been reprimanded before about her bad attitude. When she went back into the cubicle to get a history on the lady, we overheard her speaking very disrespectfully to the elderly woman. The conversation went something like this. The nurse, in a condescending voice said, "What's wrong with you?" The lady, in a weak lethargic voice said, "I don't know." The nurse said, "What do you expect me to do?" The lady said, "I hope you can find out what is wrong." "Well, you are in the wrong place sister, because we don't work magic here," stated the nurse. The elderly lady said,

"I don't like your attitude." The nurse said, "Then, you can leave." The elderly woman asked her for her cane so she could leave. This little woman was insulted. Most elderly people can't tell you what's wrong with them. All they know is that they are sick. She knew she had been disrespected. This fueled her anger. The nurse picked up her cane from the side of the cart and threw it on the bed. The elderly lady sharply said, "You didn't have to throw it!" The nursed ignored her and bent over to let the rails down so she could get out of the bed. Suddenly the nurse was grabbed by the back of her uniform jacket, and 'grandma' proceeded to beat her about the forehead with the cane. She screamed for help. The old lady said, "Don't scream now, you should have thought about this when you were being nasty!" We took our time coming because she deserved it. Even the doctor was laughing. They arrested the old lady. But 'grandma' told her, "I can sit in jail for the rest of my life! But I bet you won't get nasty with me again!"

She soon fired herself. Not long after that, one of the city court judges came into the ER. It was busy that night. He had been there for almost an hour. He called this nurse and asked her how much longer it would be before he saw the doctor? She said very impatiently, "I don't know! You must sit like everyone else and wait your turn!" The judge says, "Do you know who I am?" Her reply was, "I don't know, and I don't care." He angrily raised up out of the bed. As he started putting his clothes on, he said, "Oh, but you will." It wasn't long after that when the doctor came in to see the judge. He asked, "Where is the patient that was in this bed?" She said, "Oh, he got impatient, put his clothes on and left." Little did she know, the head administrator of the hospital was a golf buddy with the judge. Need I say more? I finally got my chance to ride with Dick. He told me all I could do was observe. I couldn't interact with any of the patients. That was good enough for me. One of the medics gave me his medic jacket to wear so I could look like the medics with the fire department. The bell went off! My first run! "Medic 40! Medic 40! 703, man down!" Shouted the dispatcher over the PA system. Go to 4700 East 5th Avenue. "703, 703, man down!" Now my adrenaline is rushing! I'm so excited! Now I get to see how the medics work in the field. I beat everyone to the ambulance. It was me, Dick, and Oscar. Oscar was Dick's partner. Oscar weighed about 160–170 pounds. He was a very handsome guy with a short neat Afro haircut and a very thin mustache. He was about 5'9" or 5'10" tall with a very pleasant personality.

When we arrived on the scene, there was a man lying on the ground near his motorcycle. Dick told Oscar to get the spine board. He was going to check the patient. I assisted Oscar. As we approached the patient, a gang of motorcycle guys pulled up. These guys looked rough. They were unshaven, long beards; and across the back of their jackets was the name of their gang. This big, stringy-haired, blond guy was obviously the leader. He asked Dick what was he doing? Dick's reply was, "This man is hurt and I'm going to take him to the hospital." We found out later that this guy was running from the motorcycle gang when he hit a slick spot and fell off his bike. The big blond guy said, "You can't take this guy anywhere. He is going with us. We have some unfinished business with him." Dick said, "Your business is going to have to wait until he gets out of the hospital, because he is going with me." The big guy says, "You don't understand. He must pay for what he did." Dick said, "I don't have anything to do with that. Oscar you and Dave put this man in the ambulance." So, while Dick and the big guy were arguing, Oscar and I put the man in the ambulance. Suddenly Dick ran to the ambulance, jumped in, and told Oscar to pull off. As we were flying down 5th Avenue to the hospital, the motorcycle gang started to chase us, shooting at the ambulance. I can't begin to tell you how afraid I was. The patient was lying on the cart, and I was lying on the floor beside him. Dick reached into his bag and pulled out his pistol. He opened the back window and started shooting at the motorcycle gang. Dick was not the kind of guy you could shoot at and not expect to get a return of fire. It was against the rules for medics to carry firearms, but Dick had his own theory. He said, "I'd rather be tried by 12 than to be carried by six." Dick always had that pistol. You never caught him without it. He said, "How you going to go to a hatchet fight, and everybody has a hatchet but you?" Oscar had radioed the police and told them we were being shot at. When the motorcycle gang heard the sirens, they immediately dispersed.

My pulse is beating extremely fast. If you thought it was fast when the call came in, you ought to take it now. This reminded me of the days of the wild, wild west. When we arrived at the hospital, I told Dick, "This really gave me a rush! Is it always like this?" Almost at the same time he and Oscar said, "This is only the beginning! You haven't seen anything yet!" Now I'm starting to second-guess myself. Do I really want to go out on the streets? Dick said, "In this city you must be ready for everything and everybody. You never know what is coming at you." As we were leaving the hospital to go back to the station, we got another call. "Medic 40! Medic 40! 709! 709! 650 Carolina." As I mentioned earlier, the medics in the field had their own code system for each emergency. Code 709 was a gunshot. After the first incident, I can honestly say I'm a little gun shy now. We arrived on the scene. Dick told me to grab the medic bag. He took the drug box. Oscar brought the bed. We went up the stairs and walked into the open door. There was a man lying on the floor, bleeding from both thighs. He says in an excited but terrified voice, "I'm glad to see you guys! I've been shot!" Suddenly, all the lights went out. A deep voice out of one of the rooms said, "If you are smart you will back out of here like you walked in." Dick immediately pulled out his pistol. He said, "We are leaving but I got my pistol in my hand. If you start firing, I'm going to start firing." The man on the floor started screaming, "Please don't leave! If you leave, they going to kill me!" But we left and went back to the rig. Oscar called the police.

The dispatcher said they were already in route. I asked Dick, "What do you do in a situation like that?" He told me something that I never forgot. He said, "Dave, you don't have to risk your life to save anyone. The most valuable life out here is yours. Who can you save if you go down? Now, you need someone to save you. Because I can't be of any use to anyone if I'm gone. My family, the public and no one else will benefit if I'm gone. They would say sure, that guy Dick was a very courageous medic. The words are fine, but they do nothing for a dead man. And the sad part is that after a few months they won't even remember your name."

The police soon arrived and arrested a lot of people. We got the guy out and took him to the hospital. Now that I've had my chance to ride, I find that I really like being in the streets. To become a medic on the streets you must be hired on the Gary Fire Department. That presented a problem to me. I had a job working for U.S. Steel full-time and I worked part-time at Lutheran General Hospital in the ER. How could I possibly work three jobs? That dilemma was soon resolved.

About a month later, I received a call from U.S. Steel asking me if I wanted to take a vacation. When I refused the vacation, I received another phone call from them stating that I was being laid off due to a reduction in the workforce. This couldn't have happened at a worse time in my life. I was recently divorced and paying child support for three children. How was I going to meet my obligations on a part-time job? My medic companions encouraged me to get a job with the fire department. In fact, they went as far as to talk to the fire chief about giving me a job as a paramedic. Because I came so highly recommended, the fire chief told me to come take a physical. I passed the physical. Then they sent me to get fitted for a uniform.

Can you imagine the faces of the people in the ER when they saw me in uniform? Not bragging, but I wore it well and I wore it proudly. This just wasn't a job for me, it was an opportunity to experience another level of my profession. I was the new "Rookie" on the streets. I wasn't new to the field of paramedics because I had plenty of experience. I was just new to the streets. The first thing I asked the EMTs with the fire department was, "Who is the best paramedic out here?" They called off three names: Dick, Delbert, and Happy. I told them "Give me six months. If I'm not better, I'll be just as good." I was really looking forward to being with Dick, but he hurt his back and was off the ambulance for a while.

I was on a mission. Like the missions on the Star Trek Enterprise, I wanted to go where no man had gone before. It wasn't long before my name was ringing throughout the department. I set those streets on fire. Because I worked in the ER and brought all my experience to the streets, they gave me the nick name Doc. Not only had I gained the respect of all the medics, but the ER doctors and nurses were also praising my work. Those years of working at Lutheran General Hospital had paid off. My diagnostic skills were so good that when I brought someone into the ER, the doctors had confidence that my clinical diagnosis was correct. Some of the paramedics would be treating patients for one problem, only to find out when they arrived at the ER, the patient had an entirely different problem. I had become so good that I could walk into the house, take one look at the patient, and just about tell you what was wrong.

I walked in the door and this man was sitting forward breathing very hard. You could hear the gurgling sound coming from his lungs. Right away I knew this man was in a condition called Pulmonary Edema. This is a condition when the heart becomes weak; the fluid backs up into the lungs and makes it almost impossible for the person to breathe. I didn't have to take my stethoscope to listen to both sides of his lungs to see if I heard bilateral rales. That's a waste of time. This person was in distress and needed emergency intervention right now. I have witnessed medics spend precious minutes listening and looking for all the cardinal signs before they start treatment. Some of these conditions I saw so many times in the ER, I didn't need to verify all those signs for treatment.

The medics I worked with were also impressed with my skills for starting IVs. As I said before, I had developed a technique where I could get an IV started with one needle stick. They were so confident in my skills, that when people would say, "I have bad veins," their first reply was, "He is only going to stick you once." And 95% of the time they were correct. I've watched medics stick people four or five times and still couldn't get the IVs started. They started calling me "One-Stick Johnson."

The medics had worked with some good guys, but I was a welcome addition to the team. I was happy to be so respected. Being new on the Gary Fire Department, I was considered a "Rookie." When you are a rookie, they treat you like a rookie. I had commanders over me now: Fire Chiefs, Station Captains, Lieutenants, and Medic Chiefs. All these paramilitary people could give me orders. If I didn't carry out the orders, there was also punishment. They could make you wash every vehicle in the station, mop and wax all the floors, wash all the walls, etc. You worked 24 hours with 48 hours off. They could make you work 48 hours with only 24 hours off if they wanted to punish you.

Some of the captains gave me a hard time, like Captain Sims. He picked at me constantly. When I came back from an ambulance run, if he saw one spot of dirt on the ambulance, he made me wash it again. I could only sit in certain places in the fire station. He would walk into the lounge and say to me, "Johnson, you can't sit in that chair. That is a captain's chair. You have to sit over there where the rookies sit." He would wait until we came in at night and say, "Johnson, you have to wash those dishes. Be sure to mop the floor and the lounge." Sometimes I would get a run before I finished. But rest assured, the job had better be finished before I got off duty the next day. This went on for a year. Now I'm not a rookie anymore. You are only a rookie for a year.

When you start out as a paramedic, they put you with one of the senior paramedics until you become proficient and learn the ropes. Guess who they put me with. Happy. That was fine. Happy was an excellent paramedic. As you recall, he was one of the reported three best. Happy had been in Vietnam. I'm not sure what happened to him over there because he refused to talk about it. He would start drinking alcohol every morning as soon as he got to work. He would drink up until noon. As I mentioned previously, once he became intoxicated, he was going to bed. It wasn't until evening that Happy came around and was able to function.

I would spend the whole morning dragging Happy around from call to call. This is how it went. When the call came in, I would go get Happy out of bed. I would put his clothes on. I would put him in the rig. Then, I would strap him in and drive to the call. If it were something I could handle by myself, I would take care of it. If I needed assistance, I would call for backup. Happy would sleep through the entire run.

One day we had a call, 701, chest pains. I did my usual, getting Happy prepared. When I got to the house, I went in alone and talked to the little elderly lady. She had experienced chest pains for about an hour. I gave her some oxygen to breathe. After taking her vitals, I wanted to start an IV. She refused. I wanted to put her on the cardiac monitor. She refused. The family convinced her to go to the hospital. She agreed to go. I told the lady that I was going to get the bed. As a paramedic, we were trained to never walk a patient with chest pain. She said, "I'll go to the hospital but I'm not getting on that bed." After exhausting all efforts by her family and myself, I agreed to do what I didn't want to do. I let her walk to the rig. She was getting so upset with us trying to convince her to get on the bed; we ran the risk of giving her a heart attack. So, I had to decide. Sometimes you can't do everything by the book. You must do what is prudent if it helps the patient. We walked her very slowly to the rig. I opened the side door to let her in. What do you think I saw? Yes, Happy had done his usual. He climbed out of the front into the back. Took off all his clothes. He had laid on the bed under the sheets and went to sleep.

I closed the door. Unable to tell them what is going on, I said, "One minute, let me get some of the equipment out of your way." I went to the back door and hit Happy on the feet. Yelling at him I said, "Get up! I have a patient!" He jumped up, slipped his pants and shirt on quickly and grabbed his shoes and crawled back into the front of the rig. I wondered for a while who was training who. I managed to get the lady to the hospital, and all was well.

When evening fell and Happy sobered up, he took a shower and put on a clean uniform. He shaved and ate. Now you were looking at an entirely different person. From about 6 p.m. on you saw a real paramedic. One evening, Happy and I received a call to go to 2675 Monroe St. 709; this is a code for a gunshot wound. When we arrived, we saw a male about 25 years old lying on the ground face up with a gunshot wound to the right side of his chest.

Happy and I jumped out and started to work on him right away. Happy was putting an IV in the patient's arm. Suddenly, this big man walked up. He was about 250 pounds and about 6'2" tall. He had a rough, mean-looking face. There was a bottle of alcohol in his hand. He took a long drink and said, "If my brother dies, I am going to kill both of you." Right at that moment the man took his last breath and did not breath again. Happy nervously looked at me. He had a very worried look on his face. In a whispering tone I said, "What do we do now?" He said, "When I count to three you run one way and I will run the other. He can only chase one of us at a time. If he chases me, you get the rig and pick me up. If he chases you, I will get the rig and pick you up. One, two, three." We jumped up and ran in different directions. He started chasing Happy. I ran to the rig, made a U-turn, and drove past him, stopping long enough for Happy to jump on the back of the rig. I made another U-turn, and we went back to get our equipment. Happy jumped off the rig, opened the back door and threw our equipment inside. This big guy was coming fast. He resembled a big rhino charging. Happy jumped in and said, "Take off!" I left there like a scared rabbit running from a wolf. I left track marks all the way to the corner. The police were just arriving and arrested the man. We called the coroner for the wounded man on the ground. Happy and I had some exciting moments. I'm so glad he was sober most of the time when we did. He was a very skilled paramedic.

A state trooper shot a man trying to flee, after he was stopped for a traffic violation. The man had some stuff on him that was going to get him arrested. He ran down the embankment off the expressway across a field. It was below 0 degrees Fahrenheit outside that day. And he was running through about three or four feet of snow. It was cold and slippery. The officer told him to halt but he kept running. The officer shot him in the leg. He didn't pursue the man. He just called us.

Upon arrival, Happy and I surveyed the area. We knew we couldn't carry the bed through three feet of snow. The man was lying about 50 yards from the expressway. We decided to carry the spine board down, put him on it and get him back to the rig. The man was about 5'8" tall and 180–190 pounds. Can you imagine trying to carry someone that heavy through snow that weighs your feet down? Each time you put your foot down you get stuck. You move one foot at a time through the field with this weight. Every time we moved; this man screamed in pain because he was shot through the femur. We finally made our way to the embankment. As we tried to climb the embankment, the patient kept sliding off the board. We asked the state trooper to give us a hand, but he refused. Happy was very angry. He said, "You should help us. You shot him." But he still refused. We decided to lay the patient in the snow, then put the spine board back in the rig and take the bed out and sit it by the door. We then tried to do a two-man carry up the hill. Finally, with much difficulty, we managed to get the man to the bed. I was so cold. I couldn't possibly assist Happy. My hands were numb. My body was so cold that I was shivering.

We put the man in the rig. He had lost so much blood that he was going into shock. Happy told me to warm up while he worked on the patient. Happy put the mast pants on this man and started an IV on him. Keep in mind, when people's limbs are cold, their veins are hard to find. Where Happy found a vein boggles my mind to this day. He said to me, "Can you drive?" I said, "I'll try." While I drove to the hospital, Happy worked on this man, vigorously trying to save his life. We got the man to the hospital safely. The doctors commended Happy for his fine work.

I commended Happy also because I was no help. He said, "Don't mention it. Sometimes you do what you have to do."

The Fire Chief knew the situation with Happy. They were also aware of what I was going through daily. He assigned me two female medics. They were Laila and Shanice. Laila was short, about 5'0" tall and thin, maybe 100 pounds. She was dark complexioned with very smooth skin. Her hair was short but neatly styled. She was a pleasant person and a good EMT. She was very streetwise. Shanice was about the same height, maybe a little taller, very shapely, with long hair, fair complexioned and very sassy. Both were very attractive ladies and good EMTs. During the day, they would ride with me. Meanwhile, Happy was back at the station doing his usual. Sleeping off whatever was bothering his soul and steeped in an alcoholic induced state of unconsciousness. I enjoyed my time with these ladies. They taught me a lot about the streets. After six months with these ladies, the Fire Chief decided I was ready to be on my own. He reassigned me to another station. I received two new partners Russ, and Lashawn. These were my partners for the next few years. Now the adventure begins.

CHAPTER 10

WORKING WITH RUSS AND LASHAWN

WORKING WITH RUSS AND LASHAWN PROVED TO be the best time I have ever had as a paramedic. We worked together for about five years, and I must say we had some adventures. There probably wasn't any combination of medics that worked together as cohesively as Russ, Lashawn, and me.

Russ was medium height, about 5'9" tall, and stocky built, with a football player's neck. His neck was so big, it looked as if his head was sitting on a tree trunk. He was also as strong as an ox. He was a very kindhearted person and very easy to get along with. He had the kind passion for helping people that I had. He was an excellent EMT. I had to always be alert around him because he was always playing jokes on me. We hit it off right from the beginning. Miss Lashawn was some kind of lady.

Lashawn was medium height and about 5'4" tall and, maybe, 150 pounds. She was very smart and a very good medic. She could stand toe-to-toe with any guy in the station. The men would pick at her all the time, but they could never top her. She could throw with the best of them. Meaning in a verbal debate, you weren't going to win. For everything you said, she had a comeback. Even when they got down and dirty, she got down and dirty with them.

She had such a quick wit. She told me she was raised with a lot of brothers, which made her very comfortable around men. It didn't matter what Russ and I threw at Lashawn, she always had something to throw back.

We just gelled. We became familiar with one another's personalities and habits. We made a great team. It didn't matter what kind of run we were on, I never had to tell them what I wanted or what to do next. They knew my every move. All I had to do was reach my hand out and whatever I wanted would be put in my hand. For example, if I were going to start an IV, they would have the IV bottle and tubing already put together and the IV line bled to get the air out. When I held my hand out, they would immediately put a tourniquet in it. When I extended my hand again, they would put the alcohol wipe in it, then the needle and then the tape. They loved to watch me start IVs because I would only stick the patient once. Anytime the patient mentioned their bad veins, they would say, "You are in luck. This guy is only going to stick you one time." Sometimes it was hard living up to that expectation. Some of those people had bad veins. Russ and Lashawn really enjoyed calling me 'Doc.' They called me 'Doc' so much I think they forgot my first name. In fact, to this very day when I see one of them, they still call me 'Doc.'

I told Russ and Lashawn that the other medics on the streets were also good. They said, "That's true but you seem to do what you do more consistently." They were always praising me. It meant something to them to get to a scene and know that things would be handled professionally and expeditiously. They said it was very frustrating to watch paramedics fumbling around, not knowing what to do, and even worse, not being able to perform their jobs. But to work with a guy that was as smooth as slicing through a piece of pie was refreshing for them.

Lashawn blended with Russ and me very well. She blended so well that she felt she should get the same treatment that Russ and I got, especially when we went to get food. Lashawn would get so frustrated with Russ and me when we went to the hospital for breakfast. We would flirt with the ladies who were serving us, especially with the cashier, which resulted in us getting our meals free. We would say very nice things to them like, "My you look so nice today." Or "I love your hair. That color really becomes you." The women would just melt. They made Lashawn pay for hers, even though she was with us. We would go to some of the Fast-food places in town and after turning on the charm; we would get all kinds of extra food and even get our meals for free. Lashawn would be so hurt. The ladies' attitudes would immediately change as soon as she came up to order. They would say in a very unprofessional tone, "Can we help you?" Russ told her if she grew a mustache, we would let her into the boy's club. I won't tell you what her reply was. But rest assured, Russ left her alone.

One morning when we got to work it seemed like "The day from hell." As soon as we arrived at work the dispatcher said, "Medic 109. Medic 109. 5275 west 38th Place. 709! 709!" 709 is gunshot wounds. Whenever we hear that code come through, we immediately start scrambling. All 709s are considered life threatening. Quick emergency intervention is needed right away. We were already in the rig. I was checking out the drugs and the equipment. Russ and Lashawn were checking the rig. So, we took off with tires screaming and sirens blasting. Russ grabbed the microphone and said, "109 is 1076. Which means, 109, our ambulance number, is in route. Once we arrived, I grabbed the drug box. Russ grabbed the bed. Lashawn grabbed the jump bag.

The door was open. We peeked inside, and as our eyes moved around the room, we saw the body of a man on the floor. The police pulled up and rushed in but stopped in their tracks. The man was in a sitting position with his body resting against the wall. The shotgun was lying across his legs. From his nose up, there was nothing there. The man had blown the entire top of his head off. We could look down into the top of his head and see fragments of the brain. Brain tissue was spattered on the wall and the ceiling. It was a gruesome sight. This was a shocking sight of a man with no eyes, no ears, just fragments of a nose. It looked as if someone had taken a knife and sliced the top of his head off. This was the first time I had seen anything like this. It made my stomach weak. I turned to the police, visibly shaken and nervous, and said, "This is a coroner's case, you don't need me." I walked out the door and went to the rig. To my surprise, Russ and Lashawn were still in the house. Most of the time, when I leave, they leave with me. I went back to the house. There they were, standing over the man. Looking inside his head discussing it as if they were two med students in an anatomy class. I said, "You sick medics! Will you please come on! Let's go!" Russ said, "What's the matter 'Doc,' you are getting squeamish?" Then he said, "Look Lashawn this is probably the medulla." I turned and walked out again. This time they followed.

As soon as we went back into service the dispatcher said, "Medic 109, medic 109 go to 725 Hovey. 709! 709!" Once again, Russ took off like he was in the Indy 500. When we arrived on the scene, there was a lady out front screaming. "My daughter has been shot! She's upstairs! She's upstairs!" We rushed upstairs. There was a young woman in her early 20s with a gunshot wound to her head. She had no obvious signs of life. The smoke was very thick in the kitchen with a strong gunpowder smell. There were large holes in the walls and the refrigerator. The mother came in and asked us if we could save her daughter. I informed her, regrettably, that the young lady was dead. She started crying and telling us what happened. The girl was dating a guy, but she had recently broken up with him. He called her on the phone and informed her that he was coming to kill her. The mother said she told her daughter to go upstairs. She, in turn, went into her dresser draw to get her gun. She had a .357 magnum. The girl called downstairs to her mother, stating that she saw the man coming towards the house with a shotgun and a pistol. He blew the locks completely out of the doors with the shotgun. Once he entered the house, the mother started shooting at him from her bedroom. He was in the kitchen shooting back. Once the mom ran out of bullets, she ran outside. This is when he went upstairs and put a bullet in the girls' head and left. The mother said repeatedly, "I told my daughter to leave that man alone because he is crazy!"

The police arrived and immediately went looking for the guy. Somehow, he just vanished. I felt so sorry for this poor woman. Being a parent, I understand how you want to try to protect your children. The mother was extremely distraught. With her head down, weeping, hopelessly saying, "If I just had some more bullets, I could have held him off." Russ and Lashawn were livid. I tried to comfort the lady as much as I could. What do you say to a person in a situation like this? What words will help the pain? We sadly collected our equipment and left.

Lashawn said, "Let's get some breakfast guys. This looks like it is going to be a long day." We went to a fast-food restaurant. This time neither Russ nor I was in the mood to put the charm on. As soon as our food came, our portable radio went off. Medic 109! Medic 109! 701! 702! 2125 Taft Street. This code was for a possible heart attack and shortness of breath. We grabbed the bag of food and ran to the rig. When we arrived at the house, we found an elderly lady sitting slumped over in a chair and she was having difficulty breathing. Russ and Lashawn immediately administered oxygen to the patient. I asked her, "How do you feel?" She said weakly, gasping for breath, "Not so good." I said, "Are you having any pain?" She said, "Yes." I said, "Are you going to let us take you to the hospital?" She said, "Not today." I took her vitals and put her on the monitor to check her EKG rhythm. Russ and Lashawn had already set up my IV. I said, "Miss, I'm going to have to start an IV on you." Her reply was, "Not today." I said, "Didn't you tell me you were having a problem breathing?" She said, "Yes." I said, "Didn't you tell me that your chest was hurting?" She said, "Yes." I said, "Are you going to let me help you?' She said, "Yes, but not today." Lashawn said, "Miss, how old are you?" She said, "86." Lashawn said, "Don't you want to live to see 87?" She said, "Sure I do, baby." I said, "You are not ready to die, are you?" She said, "Of course not." I said, "So are you going to let me help you?" Guess what she said? "Not today." We all looked at each other and started laughing.

Her daughter said, "Mother these people are here to help you." She said, "I know." Her daughter said, "Haven't they been nice and friendly to you?" She said, "They been very nice baby." The daughter said, "I thought you told me you were hurting." The little lady says, "I am baby. I'm hurting bad." The daughter said, "Then, are you going to let these nice people help you and take you to the hospital?" Russ, Lashawn, and I looked at each other and said with her in one voice, "Yes, but not today."

I explained to the daughter that we couldn't forcibly take her out of the house against her will. We suggested that she and her husband should put her in their car and take her to the hospital. We would call the hospital and let them know they were coming in. We would also follow them if they could get her to go now. The woman's husband picked the old lady up and out the house he went. I volunteered to ride with them. Guess what they said?

Not today. I'm just teasing. They said they were only three minutes from the hospital but thanks anyway. We checked on the old lady. The doctor wanted to admit her to the hospital. She agreed to stay, but not today.

As soon as we returned to the ambulance, another call came in. Medic 109! 109! Please go to 2675 Monroe Street 703, 706, stat. This is man down, drug overdose. Russ took off, telling the dispatcher that 109 was in route. We arrived on the scene knowing we had a drug overdose victim in the house. Russ and Lashawn knew what I was going to do. Russ grabbed the bed and the spine board. Lashawn grabbed the jump bag. I had the defibrillator and the drug box. When we entered the house, a young lady met us at the door. She was screaming. "They are not breathing! My husband and his friend are not breathing!" In front of us were two men lying on the floor, face up, with syringes still imbedded in their arms? They appeared to be in their late 20s, and both were about 5'9" tall and very muscular. Both men had beards, but they were trimmed very neatly. I immediately did a quick assessment. I found both men with very labored breathing and both were non-responsive to verbal or painful stimuli.

Russ and Lashawn knew exactly what I had to do. We had a drug in our drug box, Narcan. This drug is a drug antagonist. It will reverse the effects of most drug overdoses immediately. Since both men were in severe respiratory distress, and the drug has almost completely suppressed their respiratory drive, we had to work quickly. I put an airway in both men and Russ was jumping back and forth, bagging both men. I didn't have time to start the IVs. I decided to put the tourniquet on their arms and administer the drug right into their veins. This is what I like about Russ and Lashawn. I didn't have to tell them to give me a tourniquet. They had already put the tourniquet around the arms of both men. They had also taken the Narcan out of the drug box and had it ready for me to administer.

Then, 30 seconds after I administered the drug to the first man, he started to come around. I told Russ to bag him until he became fully aroused. Bagging is the process of forcing air or oxygen into their lungs with a bag valve. We did the same to the other man with the same results. We really felt good. We had just saved these two men. The men weren't 100% alert yet, but they were coming around. I started IVs on both men and gave them some more Narcan. The young lady told us that they had shot up Heroin. This is a very powerful drug and is not easily neutralized. It depends on the amount they took and the quality of the drug.

The men came around. Both men were able to stand on their own. They asked us why we started IVs on them? I explained to them that we were trying to save their lives and that they were almost gone. One of the men walked up to me, looked me right in the face and said, "Do you know what you just did?" I said, "Yes I just saved your life." He said, "No you bleep! Bleep! You just messed up my high! It took us all night to get enough money to get high and you just killed it in a few minutes." Russ said, "Hey man, we just saved your life." He said, "I don't recall calling you to do anything." Lashawn said, "You couldn't call us. Your wife called." He turned and grabbed his wife and said, "Why did you call these people? I do this all the time and you know it." Shaking and crying she said, "I thought you were going to die." He said, "Then you should have let me die! But now you and these people have messed up our high and somebody is going to pay." The other guy said, "You might as well start coming out of your pockets because no one is leaving until we get enough money to get some more drugs." Lashawn said, "I'm not giving you nothing! Next time we'll let you die, you ungrateful bleep, bleep." I said, "Lashawn be quiet." Then Russ cranked up. He said, "I wish you would try to take something from me. You are going to get more than a needle in your arm. I saved your life, and you want to rob us and threaten us?" I said, "Be cool Russ." The one thing about a heated situation is someone must keep a cool head. I knew my crew was always ready for battle. Being the Chief Medic in the field makes me not only responsible for my life, but the lives of my medics. I said to the guy, "Hey man just calm down." He yelled at me with all he had, "I DIDN'T CALL YOU! Now unless you are prepared to die, I suggest you go into your pockets and give me some money." Russ and Lashawn immediately said, almost at the same time, "I'm not giving you anything, so I guess we are going to have to fight." Then they grabbed their IVs and pulled them out of their arms.

I see the situation is escalating very fast. Somebody is probably going to get hurt very bad. I was trying to think fast as to what we could do, but a way out was made for us. The police came. They generally respond to drug overdoses, but they had been delayed because they were on another call. Once they walked in, it was obvious to them that a fight was about to break out. The police said, "What's going on?" I told him, "These guys had shot up heroin and were almost dead. Now that we have them back, they want to fight us and take our money." This really made these two men mad. They started yelling and cursing and getting in our faces. The policemen grabbed them, and a big fight broke out! Russ, Lashawn, and I helped the police subdue these men. They were arrested and taken to jail. Sometimes it is good to assist the police. Just think what would have happened if they had overpowered the police? Yes, these guys would have killed everyone. I think what really sent them over the edge was knowing that they weren't going to get any money or drugs, and the high that they had was all they were going to get. But now that's gone.

As we walked back to the rig Russ said, "I hate the police came 'Doc' because the guy that was in my face was about to get knocked out." I said, "What about the guy in my face Russ? I don't have the knockout punch." He said, "Lashawn and I were going to go and cook some popcorn and laugh ourselves to death watching you running from that guy." I said, "Russ, I assumed that you would have helped me." He said, "I knocked out one guy, 'Doc.' Do I have to get Lashawn to knock the other one out?" Lashawn cranked right up. She says with this brave, I don't take any stuff demeanor, "You see they didn't get in my face."

We laughed it off as we were getting in the rig. Russ put us back in service. "Medic 109 is 10-8." This means that you are finished with one run and ready for another. Before we could pull off the dispatch said, "109! 109! Ridge and Grant! Ridge and Grant! 711! 711! This is a car accident. The dispatcher said over the air, "The car has been hit by a train." We took off. As you can see, we haven't had a break yet. While in route to serious runs, we always discuss our plan of action. We decide at that point who's going to get what and who's going to do what. When we arrived, there were medics from another ambulance service on the scene. This happens many times. It all depends on who called in the run. There were other ambulance services in the city. There was also a female county police on the scene. The train had pushed the car about 30–40 feet up the track. I immediately asked the other medics if any of them were paramedics? They said, "No we are EMTs." This run was going to require advanced life support. The EMTs on the scene couldn't provide that kind of support. I immediately took over the scene. If there had been a paramedic with them, I would have assisted if they needed it, or just went on my way. On exam, I found a woman in her 50s in the driver's seat. She was the only passenger. She was alert but the steering wheel was pushed in on her chest. It had her pinned against the seat. She was experiencing respiratory difficulty. Her color was pale. Her skin was cool and moist. Her blood pressure was 90/60 and her pulse was 140. This tells me that this woman is possibly bleeding internally. She could have fractured ribs that possibly punctured a lung. She could also have a ruptured spleen or a lacerated liver. The fire rescue squad was busy trying to pry the steering wheel off her chest. I started an IV of ringers lactate. The other medics had already put oxygen on the woman. I told Russ to bring the spine board and the bed. Lashawn helped him carry it down the tracks. The firemen pulled the whole top half of the car back, which pulled the steering wheel back. Once the pressure was off her chest, she screamed with pain! We put a collar around her neck. One of the medics from the other service said, "Excuse me sir, but this is our patient." I responded, "This patient needs advanced life support. There is not a paramedic with you to give her that, so I'm going to have to take her."

They said, "But we were here first." This is when the female county police officer spoke up and said, "You just can't come in here and take their patient. They were here before you got here." Russ spoke up before I could say a word, "You don't have anything to do with this case. Your job is to just direct traffic." I said, "Russ let me handle this." My reply was, "Officer, I don't have time to debate this issue with you. This lady needs medical attention right away. These medics aren't equipped to give her the attention she needs." She said, "Sir, you are out of line." My reply was, "I don't know enough about your job to give you advice as to what you are supposed to do. You don't know enough about this job to give me advice. So, I suggest you allow us to take care of this woman and leave." She says, "I can arrest you." My response was "If you do, I will press charges against you for interfering with a paramedic while on duty. You will be lucky to get a job as a crossing guard after that." Now Russ and Lashawn cranked up again. I yelled at them, "Stay focused, we need to save this woman! You don't have time to argue with this officer. Let's get her out and go!" I told the other medics, "If you want to assist us you can. Otherwise please stand back." We extricated her out to the spine board and away we went.

We weren't pulling rank just to pull rank. Most ambulance services rely on runs to get revenue. The more runs they take, the more money they can get. Sometimes the patient gets caught in this political triage. What is more important, giving the patient the best care? Or the money? This lady was escalated to a class three trauma and was immediately taken to surgery. Our intervention with her getting fluids possibly saved her life. If she had gone with them, with no advanced intervention she might have died. By the time she got to the hospital, her shock would have been so advanced, they couldn't have reversed it.

It is well past noon now. We never got breakfast, and everyone is hungry. We stopped at Kentucky Fried Chicken. Before we could swallow the first bite of food, the dispatcher said, "Medic 109! Medic 109! 711! 711! 29th and Clark Road." This is another car accident. Picture someone trying to eat while an ambulance is speeding. Russ hit the brakes because someone pulled in front of him. The food and drinks started flying. Lashawn's drink flew up in the air and landed on her head. The potatoes that I was eating were now all over my face because I was thrown forward into the container. The potatoes are hot! I'm trying to get hot potatoes off my nose! Lashawn is frantic because her hair is wet! As we continued to speed, she tried to compose herself and get a towel to dry her face and head. We both looked at Russ, we were so angry. Russ was laughing so hard. He paid us no attention as we yelled at him. Lashawn was cursing him in every language she knew.

We arrived on the scene, and it is ugly. Two cars met head on just as they crossed over the bridge at Clark Road. This is a small two-lane street. One of the cars was trying to pass another car at a high rate of speed and misjudged the distance of the approaching car. They were young teenaged males. The driver of the speeding car was thrown completely through the windshield. He was lying 15-20 feet in front of his car on the side of the road. He was killed on impact. His face was smashed in. He had deep cuts on his forehead and on the side of his neck. His body was twisted with the legs going one way and the torso going another. The passenger in his car was also dead. His head was stuck in the windshield. The impact was so great that he broke the seat. Being strapped to the seat by the seat belt kept him from going out the window. But his head was on the opposite side of the window. The force probably broke his neck or severely injured the brain.

The other car that was hit had four people in it, two men and two women. They were middle-aged married couples on their way to a wedding. One of the couple's daughters was getting married. The people in the back seat were in the trunk. The car was smashed like an accordion. The two in the front seat were in the back and the engine was sitting on top of them. It took more than an hour to cut these people out of the wreckage. They were killed on impact. It was obvious that they died from crushing injuries. There was blood everywhere. Pieces of the car had impaled those in the back seat. The engine practically covered the couple in the front. All we could see was their heads. The officer on the scene said, "This is one of the worst I have witnessed." We stood there frozen in our tracks, feeling helpless. Cars can become deadly missiles in the wrong hands. We slowly walked back to the rig. Everyone was silent. We went back in service. Strangely, we didn't get a run right away. Once we arrived at the station, Russ went to the bunkroom and laid down on his bed. Lashawn went to the female quarters. I went into the kitchen to get something to drink.

Suddenly, a lady ran across the street to the station. She was pounding on the door, screaming at the top of her voice, "Come quick! Someone come quickly! My baby has been hit by a car! My baby has been hit by a car!" Russ, Lashawn, and I responded at the same time. We jumped into the rig and drove across the street. We jumped out of the rig. On the ground, lying face down, was a four-year-old boy. He was bleeding from a cut on his forehead. We noticed that he wasn't breathing. We immediately started CPR. Lashawn opened my intubation kit and gave me the intubation tube. I got the tube in on the first try. We put the baby on a spine board, put him in the ambulance and away we went. His mom rode in the front seat of the ambulance. I put the baby on the monitor. I called the hospital to notify them of what we had. The baby was in a Sinus Tach rhythm. (A very rapid heart rhythm). As we bagged him, he started to breath on his own and fight the tube. We arrived at the hospital. They took the baby to the trauma room. He suffered head injuries, but survived. The doctor came to us and said, "Good job men. If it wasn't for your quick intervention, this child would be dead." The mother hugged us, repeatedly thanking us. The other family members and the neighbors came to the hospital to see about the baby. We were told that while playing, the other children were chasing this little one. To keep from being caught, he ran into the street.

When they were informed that the baby was going to be ok, they all let out a big yell. We walked out to the rig to put our equipment in it. They ran outside to congratulate us. We were treated like heroes.

This is the part of the job that is rewarding. It means a lot to be able to give loved ones back to their families. We would have loved to have been able to help those people in that head on collision. Even though you feel empathy for the people, you can't carry one run to the next. Irrespective of the situation or circumstances we encounter, we must stay focused for the next run.

Our break was short lived. Once we went in service the dispatcher gave us another run. Medic 109! Medic 109! 35th and Broadway! 35th and Broadway! 709! 709. This is a gunshot wound. Ordinarily we would not have to take a run on the opposite end of town. Each ambulance covered a certain district. But if everyone else is already on a run, you must cover that area if a run comes in. Russ said, "Ok, 'Doc' and Lashawn hang on. I'm going to have to step on it." You see, response time is critical when people are bleeding. The trauma surgeons refer to these situations as the golden hour. If you can get the patient transported to the hospital so they can get the patient in surgery within one hour, they have a good chance of survival.

One of the problems we had was that our rigs were old. They broke down a lot. We arrived on the scene. Here is a man lying face up on the floor with a gunshot wound to the abdomen. He was of Latin descent. He looked to be in his early 30s. The man was about 6'0" tall and maybe 170 pounds. His intestines were protruding out of his abdomen, and he was bleeding profusely. Russ and Lashawn were the best. They already had an IV set up in the rig. The spine board was already on the bed. The monitor was already open and set up. We rushed in. The first thing we did was put a sterile, moist stomach dressing on his abdomen. Then we rolled him over on the spine board, put him on the bed, and out to the rig we went. I took my scissors and cut his clothes to check for other possible sites of injury. Always undress your patient. The first time you don't, you will miss something. I had one man that was shot in the thigh. I didn't take his shirt off. What puzzled me was why he went into shock so fast. When we arrived at the hospital and took his clothes off, they found a bullet wound in his back. From that point on, I always undressed gunshot wounds. I told Russ to take off. I would do everything in route.

Russ drove to the corner. He stopped at the stoplight and the rig went dead. He tried to start it back but there was no response. Now we have a real problem. I have a trauma patient in the rig with a gunshot wound to the belly and no way to transport him to the hospital. Russ was so mad. He got out, slammed the door, and kicked the rig.

I called the dispatcher. I told him, "I need assistance stat." He said, "All the rigs are out on runs." I said, "Send me a fire engine." He did. We took the patient out of the rig, opened the back door of the engine, and put him in it. The firemen jumped on the back and away we went. Russ stayed with the rig. Lashawn and I went to the hospital. I called and told them that I was coming in on a fire engine so clear the ramp. Fortunately, we got the man there safely and he survived.

Lashawn and I waited at the hospital for Russ. He had to go to the main station to get a spare rig. One of the medics at the hospital took us to the main station.

The mechanics always kept at least two rigs in the station for spares. We had some real characters working at these stations. They can become very creative when needed. The Chief Medic told us to take the rig up front. As we walked toward the rig a call came in for us. Medic 109! Medic 109! Go to 2253 Connecticut. There is a house fire with people inside. We ran to the rig, hopped in, and took off.

We were no more than 50-feet from the station when we heard someone beating on the window in the back of the rig. We stopped the rig and looked in the back window. There was Fat Freddy, nude in the back of the rig, with a woman. He was whispering, "Take me back. Take me back."

Russ stopped the rig, made a U-turn, and went back to the station. He pulled up on the ramp with the siren and lights flashing. Everyone came out to see what the problem was. Out of the side door jumps Fat Freddy with a sheet over him and the woman was right behind him. The guys were lying on the ground from laughter. Russ was fussing away. He said, "I'm sick of these guys using these rigs for their hotel." Lashawn said, "Do you guys know who the woman was? I'm going to tell Fat Freddy's wife unless he pays me."

We get on the scene of the fire. There are three children trapped in the house. The mother is standing outside screaming, "My babies! My babies!" The firemen brought the first baby out. He looked to be three or four years old. The child was on fire. His legs and arms were smoking. Lashawn grabbed the baby and started giving him mouth to mouth. The firemen came out with another child. He appeared to be about 12 years old. He was burned very badly. All his clothing was burned off. He was coughing and choking. Another ambulance pulled up with a paramedic. I told them to take this child to the hospital stat. The firemen couldn't find the last child. I intubated the baby, and we took off to the hospital.

Lashawn was crying as she was doing chest compressions. The baby was unconscious and without a heartbeat. The more we worked on the baby the harder Lashawn cried. She had a child about this baby's age. We got the baby to the hospital. The staff worked on the baby, but the child died. This was a beautiful child. Though she was three or four years old, she appeared so tiny, and Lashawn worked so hard to keep her alive. She laid there with her eyes closed. She had a thick head of hair, and long eyelashes with a beautiful complexion. The whole staff was in tears.

The mother was just getting off work when she arrived home to find her house on fire. We later learned that they found a male's body in the house. The mother had left the children with her 22-year-old brother. He was babysitting. He had been drinking and fell asleep with a cigarette in his hand. This set the couch on fire causing this situation. Losing children is never easy. It's hard to keep your composure.

We wrote our report. We expressed our sympathy to the mother and went back in service. The dispatcher gave us another run. 109! Go to 4506 East 21st Avenue. 706! 706! This is the code for a drug overdose. While in route, LaShawn was composing herself. The apartment that we were going to was in the Housing Projects. The door was open. There was a man at the top of the stairs. He said, "The lady you are looking for is up here." We found a female about 30 years old lying on a bed and unresponsive to verbal or painful stimuli. The man told us she had overdosed on drugs, but he wasn't sure which ones they were. She had three small children sitting on a bed with no sheet on it. The oldest appeared to be five or six years old. The youngest was maybe one year old. The oldest child was holding the youngest child. The children were minimally dressed. The baby had on a disposable diaper. The other children only had on pants with no top or shoes. There were two other men in the house who looked drugged out.

We started an IV on the woman and gave her Narcan. She was still not responsive. We knew we were going to have to take her to the hospital. The problem was what do we do with the children. We couldn't leave the children there with the other addicts. We inquired of the neighbors, but no one wanted to get involved. We contacted the police, who took the children with them. The other men in the apartment told us they thought she might have shot some bad heroin. It is sad to see the environment that some of these children are raised in.

The hospital called protective services. They took the children away from the woman until she cleaned up her life.

It is night, about 10 p.m. We have been running all day. Everyone is tired and hungry. But, as soon as we get back to the station, the dispatcher gave us another run. 109! 109! 5th and Broadway! 5th and Broadway! 709 to the face! It is amazing the energy you muster for the urgent runs. We rushed to the rig and took off! What we saw on arrival still haunts me to this day. I'm sure many people have seen horror movies, but none could compare to this man's injury. Here is a man walking around with no face, screaming as loud as he can. Russ pulled right up to him in the rig. When he turned and looked at us, we all screamed. This man was shot with a shotgun in a drive-by shooting. The blast took the front of his face completely off. Picture this: All we see is bone, shaping the eye sockets where eyes should be. There is no nose, nor mouth or chin; just fragments of teeth with the upper and lower jawbone visible. There was bloody skin and tissue hanging from the face area. The blood vessels were squirting blood across the face or what was left of it. The frightening part was that this man was still talking. He said, "They shot my face off! They shot my face off!" Can you imagine a skeleton talking to you?

We identified ourselves and put the man in the rig. We couldn't keep him still to do anything for him. I told Russ to drive to the hospital as fast as he could. I radioed ahead to the hospital and told them to be prepared for a gruesome sight. On arrival, we put a towel over the man's face. When the nurses took the towel away, they started screaming and running. The man set up and told the doctor, "They shot my face off." The doctor was frozen in his tracks.

The man had rendered him speechless. This poor man said a few more words, then he fell back on the bed and expired.

Russ, Lashawn, and I agreed that we needed a drink. We drove back to the station. We were very tired. Lashawn went to her room. Russ and I went to the bunkroom and just fell across our beds. But five minutes later the dispatcher says, "109! 109! 1021 Noble! 703, man down!" Russ and I got up, dragging to the rig. Lashawn didn't respond. I beat on her door and said, "Come on Lashawn, we have a run." She said," I'm sorry 'Doc' but I can't make it." Russ and I pulled off. When we arrived on the scene, we found a middle-aged man lying face down on the floor. We could smell the alcohol on him. I asked his wife what was wrong with him. She said, "He came home drunk and fell on the floor." I examined him and found no obvious injuries. I asked his wife if she wanted us to take him to the hospital. She said, "No I just called you guys to get him up and put him in bed. He's too heavy for me to handle by myself." Russ said in a very exasperated voice, "Ma'am are you aware that this is an emergency ambulance service? Why didn't you call a neighbor or a relative?" The lady said, expressing irritation, "I couldn't get anyone, so I called you." Russ said, "You still have a problem because this is not an emergency. We don't come out of the fire station to get drunks off the floor and put them in bed." The lady said, "What am I supposed to do with him? I just can't leave him on the floor." I said, "Come on Russ, let's put the man in bed." Russ, in a very frustrated voice, said, "Doc this is not an emergency." I said, "I know Russ. Since we are here, let's put him in bed. The sooner we do. The sooner we can leave."

We went back to the station. We both crawled to our beds. After about 15 minutes we got another call. "109! 109! 2576 Hamlin! 713!" That is a code for an unknown emergency. Russ immediately got up and went around to the passenger's door. I said, "Where are you going Russ? Who's going to drive?" He said, "Doc I'm too tired to drive. You will have to drive this time." I drove to the scene. Once we went inside of the house. We encountered a young lady whose six-year-old son had a small cut on his index finger. I said, "Ma'am is this the only problem?" She said, "Yes, my son cut his hand." I said, "When did he cut it?" She said, "He cut it this morning." Russ just turned and walked out the door. She said, "Where is he going?" I said, "Ma'am, this is not a true emergency. If you wanted it treated, why didn't you take him to the hospital this morning?" She said, "I was at work when he did it." "So, why do you think you need an ambulance for a small cut on a finger?" I asked. Her reply was, "My car is out of gas, and I don't have any money. So, are you going to take me to the hospital or not?" I said, "Come on." I took her to the hospital. Russ never got out of the rig. We went back to the station.

Within five minutes the dispatcher gave us another run. I'm so sleepy now I know I can't drive. Russ said, "Doc, I can't make it." I called the dispatcher over the telephone. I asked him, "Can you give this run to someone else so that we can get a little rest? We are both too tired to drive." He agreed.

We both fell asleep right away. Suddenly, the dispatcher comes over the air, "109! 109! 2560 Harrison! Sick baby! Sick baby!" I looked at my watch and only 10 minutes have passed. Russ said, "Doc, I thought he was going to let us rest." I said, "I did too." We crawled to the rig. Russ tried to drive. We finally arrived on the scene. We went into the house. I asked the lady what the problem was. She said, "My six-year-old daughter has a cold." Russ became belligerent. He said, "It's 2 a.m. in the morning. Is this what you called us for?" It was obvious that sleep deprivation was getting to Russ. He had lost his patience. I said, "Russ go to the rig, I'll handle it." I explained to her that colds are not emergencies unless the child is having respiratory difficulty. I examined the child and found no obvious distress. I asked her why she wanted to go to the ER? She said, "Because the child keeps crying and won't stop coughing." I said, "How long has the child had a cold?" She said, "For about a week." It was obvious that once again we were on a non-emergency run. Some people don't understand what constitutes an emergency. They use the ambulance for their personal cab. I took her to the rig and to the hospital. Once again, Russ did not get out of the rig.

We slowly drove back to the station. I was driving and Russ was the passenger. The lights would change to green. The horns from the cars behind us would start to blast. I woke up realizing I had fallen asleep at the wheel. Slowly I took my foot off the gas and tried to steer us safely to the station. This went on at every red light. Finally, we made it to the station. We went in, fell across the bed, and went fast asleep.

Suddenly I heard the bell go off. I said, "Come on Russ we got a run." Russ said, "Doc I didn't hear anything." I said, "Get your lazy self-up, Russ. Let's go." As we went slowly to the rig, he stated again, "Doc I didn't hear anything." I climbed under the wheel and said in a slurred voice, "Medic 109 is 1076, which means in route. The dispatcher came back and said, "1076 to where 109?" I said, "Didn't you call us?" He said, "No." Russ got out of the rig saying in a tired slow voice, "I told you didn't nobody call us, Doc." We went back to bed. We both fell into a deep sleep.

Once again, I heard the bell go off. I said, "Come on Russ we got a run." He said slowly and deliberately, "Doc no one called us. I didn't hear anything." I said, "You were sleeping too hard Russ. They just called us." We crawled to the rig again. I said, "109 is 1076." The dispatcher came back and said, "1076 to where 109."

Russ got out and slammed the door as he walked away saying, "Doc, I could kill you!" We went back to bed again.

After a brief period, I heard the bell again. I said, "Come on Russ, I heard the bell again." The other guys in the bunkroom said, "Russ, why don't you hit him in the head and put him out for the rest of the night so we can all get some sleep?"

We were so tired from running all day and into the night that I was hallucinating. I was hearing calls in my sleep. This job can really wear a man out. We didn't get any more calls that night, which was good.

The next morning, we were laughing about the phantom calls I heard. Lashawn said, "I didn't mean to abandon you guys, but I would have been worthless."

Was it the night from hell? No. It was the shift from hell! We had many nights like that one.

The highlight of my career came the very next workday. When we arrived for work, everyone seemed to be in a good mood. It is amazing what a little rest will do for you. The Medic Chief called me on the phone. He told me the Fire Chief informed him that the Vice President of the United States, George H. W. Bush was coming to U.S. Steel. They are the largest steel makers in the country. They had just finished building a new continuous caster. This would allow them to pour steel in a continuous cycle, which would increase their production. The Vice President was invited to give the dedication speech.

His staff said they needed an ambulance service in their entourage for emergency purposes. The Fire Chief told the Chief Medic to pick his best men for the job. We got the call. We were told to get our best uniforms and come down to the main station for a briefing with the FBI. They can't allow anyone near the Vice

President without a thorough background check first. When I informed Russ and Lashawn, they were so excited.

We cleaned up our rig. It was spotless. We put on our best uniforms and went to the number one station. The FBI asked us numerous questions. Once we cleared with them, they instructed us to go to the Gary Airport and wait for the Vice President's plane. Naturally, Russ wanted to drive.

When we arrived at the airport all the roads were closed off. There were policemen everywhere. The FBI briefed us on the ambulance's position in the motorcade. Shortly, the plane landed. We had the opportunity to see Air Force One. It was a huge plane. Once the plane landed, they rolled the steps up to the door. The door opened suddenly. Our hearts were pounding with excitement. Our faces dawned smiles from ear to ear. The Vice President's staff emerged first. Then suddenly we saw the figure of a man that appeared to be the Vice President. The blur of his movement made it impossible for us to be sure of what we were experiencing. The security was so tight that they moved him swiftly down the stairs and into a limousine. Russ said, "Here we go Doc!" I said, "Stay with him Russ, we are the Vice President's personal medics."

Our ambulance was positioned about six vehicles behind the Vice President's limo. They took him on a specifically mapped route to the caster. On arrival, the secret service took him in judiciously. As we were getting out of the rig, one of the Agents said, "You guys can just wait in the rig. If we need you, we will come and get you." We were disappointed when he said that. We really wanted to go inside.

Russ and Lashawn looked at me. Russ said, "Doc we are supposed to be the Vice President's personal medics. If someone shoots him in there, by the time they get to us the man could be dead." Lashawn said, "We need to be right where he is. If something happens, we can be right on top of it. You are the paramedic in charge. So, what are you going to do?" I said, "You are right! We're going in!" I told Russ to get the Bio-com (our radio to the hospital). I told Lashawn to get the jump bag and I would carry the drug box.

We approached the door. The agent said, "Where are you going?' I said, "I'm paramedic Johnson and these are my assistants. We are the Vice President's personal medics." We can't affectively assist him way out here. We need to be close enough so that if he sneezes, we can be right on it. If something happens to him, I'm going to tell my superiors that you were responsible for detaining us. He thought for a minute and said, "Come on in but don't get in the way." Russ and Lashawn broke out with big smiles.

As we walked in, we noticed there were chairs set up for the audience. There were tables set up buffet style with a food spread from one end to the other. All of Gary's big politicians were there. Some of the well-known ministers were also present. Russ said, "I see why they didn't want us to come in Doc. Look at all that food." Lashawn said, "Doc are we going to eat?" Being pumped up, now my reply was, "Sure we are," as I stuck my chest out. "We are a part of the Vice Presidents entourage."

We ate and ate and ate. After we finished, Russ said, "Hey Doc, why are we here in the back. We should be up front. If something happens to the man, we will have to wade through all these people to get to him." I said, "You are right Russ, let's move up front." Keep in mind, not only were there people sitting, but there were people standing. The place was full. So, we grabbed our equipment and started moving through the crowd toward the front.

There were Secret Service men in the ceiling, sitting on beams and observing everything. They had earpieces in their ears, constantly talking or communicating with one another. The closer we go to the front the more they seemed to talk. Once we reached the front, I turned around and there were agents all around us. One agent pulled back his jacket and showed me an Uzi (a rapid-fire machine gun). He said sternly, "What are you doing?" My reply was, "We are the Vice President's personal medics, and we were trying to get closer to him." He said, "Do you see those men in the ceiling? Their job is to alert us to any strange movement here on the floor. We were told that there were two men and a lady with bags in their hands moving toward the front. You guys could have gotten shot. You can't go anywhere near that man without clearance." I said, "We have on uniforms. Why would you suspect us?" His reply was, "Someone could easily masquerade as a medic, policeman, press agent, etc. We must watch everyone. So, you guys stay right here until it's over."

I whispered to Russ, "You're about to get us shot." The man said, "Don't move." And we didn't move a muscle. We were almost afraid to breathe. When they finished, they whisked him out like they brought him in. We were told to go back to our rig. We followed the entourage to Air Force One. They briskly took him to the plane and away they went.

We left and went back to the station. It was an interesting experience, one that really shook us up. But after it was over, we managed to have a big laugh over it. We were passing the blame as to who was responsible for getting us in trouble. We all agreed that trying to go through the crowds with our bags did make us look suspicious. But it was an honor to be selected to be a part of the Vice President's motorcade. This just shows you the kind of confidence our Chief had in us.

Working with Russ and Lashawn was probably the most fun I have had on any job. Russ was always playing jokes on me. There was one fireman that was always in a bad mood. Most of the guys stayed out of his way. Russ and I had just come in off a run. It was hot outside and I wanted something cold. As I looked in the refrigerator, I saw some ice cream. I yelled to Russ asking, "Whose ice cream is this?" He said, "You want some?" as if it belonged to him. I said, "Yes." He said, "Help yourself." I tried to eat as much as I could because Russ was always trying to eat all my good stuff.

The bad-spirited fireman came in from a fire and went to the refrigerator to get his ice cream. He opened the box and saw most of it was gone. He yelled angrily, "Who ate my ice cream?" Imagine how I felt. Sitting there with a mouth full of ice cream and it also running down my chin. I looked at Russ and he was falling down laughing. I said, "Russ, "I thought this was your ice cream?" He said, "Doc, I just asked if you wanted some. I never said it was mine."

I tried my best to explain to this guy what happened. He walked out and slammed the door. I said, "Come on Russ I got to go buy this guy some more ice cream." He was laughing so hard he was in tears.

Then there was the time we had just received new rigs. Russ wanted to drive, and I wanted to drive. When a run came in, Russ beat me to the driver's seat. After we took the patient to the hospital, I sat down and did my report. When I finished, I looked around to see where Russ was. He was at the nurse's station talking with the nurses. I said to myself this is perfect. I eased out to the rig hoping he wouldn't notice me. Russ would have no choice but to let me drive.

I got behind the wheel and waited for Russ to come out. I knew I had got him. He came to my door and said, "Hey Doc, the dispatcher wants to speak to you on the Red Phone." (This is a phone in the hospital ER where the dispatcher could reach us directly if we were out of the rig.) I was so disgusted that he would call me now.

I went inside, picked up the phone and said, "Paramedic Johnson." All I heard was a dial tone. I said to myself, "There is no one on this phone." I ran back to the rig and there was Russ sitting behind the steering wheel laughing for all he was worth. I just went to the other side and got in. He said, "Doc you are so easy. I can get you whenever I get ready. I saw you run outside. I told the nurses to watch this. He will be right back."

Russ seemed to enjoy setting me up. We had such a good time together. Coming to work was a pleasure. Each turn had its own adventures and there were no two alike. If I had to do it all over again, I'd do it without hesitation. We had so many adventures. I just can't remember them all.

I worked with Russ and Lashawn for five years. Russ applied and was accepted by the state police. I told him that they would have to cut out a peach basket to make him a hat. The others wouldn't be big enough. He soon left the fire department.

Lashawn went back to school to become a paramedic. I assisted her. She was the first female paramedic with the department. Later she received her own crew.

I received another crew. I truly missed Russ and Lashawn. After they left things were never the same. The chemistry that we had was never duplicated. I worked with many crews but the only ones that came close to Russ and Lashawn were Stock and Paulette.

One book is not enough to tell you about my many experiences as a paramedic. However, what I have shared are some of my most memorable moments from *THE SIRENS NEVER STOP!*

WHERE ARE THEY NOW?

I have had the pleasure of working with some interesting people. I am sure that their lives have taken different paths. To my knowledge this is what has happened to them:

1.	Mrs. Livingston,	She retired many years ago.
2.	Mrs. Draper,	She worked her way up to the Assistant VP Position at Lutheran General.
3.	Sam,	He moved back to Chicago, Illinois.
4.	Dick	He was Asst Director of Emergency Services. Not sure what he is doing now.
5.	Ned	He finally retired last year from the ER. He had almost 40 years of service.
6.	Dr. Westano	He left the ER years ago. He is probably retired now.
7.	Dr Mesta	He is still an ER doctor at one of the area hospitals.
8.	Miss Sills,	She left the ER years ago. Not sure where she is now.
9.	Irene	She left Lutheran General. She probably married Mike, her boyfriend who worked in surgery.

10.	Sherri,	She got married and moved to California.
11.	Oscar	He is a Fire Department dispatcher now.
12.	Betty,	She quit to start a modeling career.
13.	Gerald	He is the director of Emergency Physicians.
14.	Mrs. Aaronson,	She became House Supervisor.
15.	Happy	He went back to school for nursing and became a RN.
16.	Herman,	He died years ago.
17.	Eddie,	He became sick and passed away.
18.	Fred,	He retired from the Fire department and moved away.
19.	Harold	He also retired from the Fire department. He is working part-time as a paramedic.
20.	Laila,	She quit years ago not sure what she is doing now.
21.	Shanice	She quit and acquired a job at the local Post Office.
22.	Stock	He quit and moved out of town.
23.	Paulette	She is carrying the torch. She is one of the few remaining members of our old crew that is still on the ambulance crew.
24.	Russ	He is a State Trooper. We are still best friends.
25.	Lashawn,	She went to school for nursing and now is working as a nurse.
25.	Yours Truly	Well, let's say I'm **FULLY RETIRED**!!!

ABOUT THE AUTHOR

Mr. David Johnson retired in October 2003 and still lives in Dallas, Texas. He is married and has four children. His hobbies are fishing and traveling.

Mr. Johnson went to school and worked in Gary, Indiana for the past 34-plus years. During that time, he wore two employment hats for 20 years. He worked at United States Steel and with the Gary Fire Department as a paramedic.

Mr. Johnson graduated from Ivy Tech with a degree in Office Administration and a Certificate in Medical Coding and Billing. He also went to Purdue University for Nursing. Mr. Johnson was certified in all special areas in being a paramedic.

Medicine has and will always be a passion of Mr. Johnson, but he wants to get involved in an area that is not as stressful as being a paramedic.

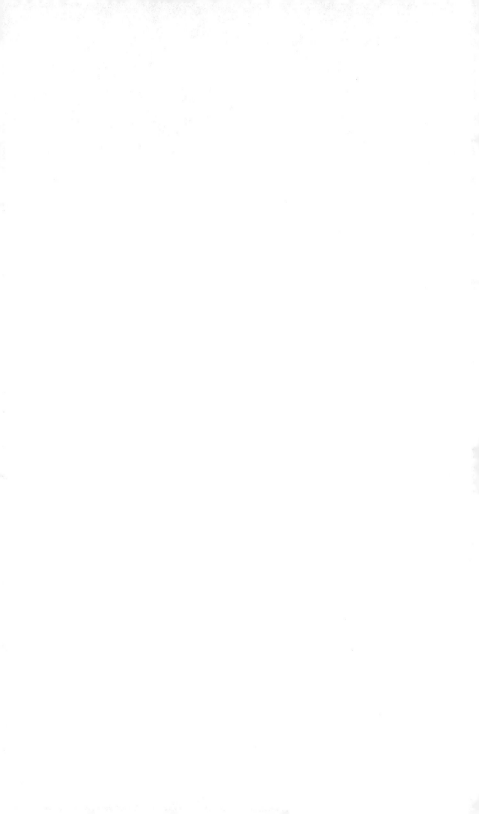